Miracle Healing Power through Nature's Pharmacy

Miracle Healing Power through Nature's Pharmacy

William L. Fischer

Fischer Publishing Corporation
Canfield, Ohio 44406

Miracle Healing Power through Nature's Pharmacy

ISBN: 0-915421-04-6

Library of Congress Catalog Number: 85-081689

Printed in the United States of America

TABLE OF CONTENTS

Table of Contents (continued)

Dedication

Considering the toxic side-effects of most of the pharmaceutical drugs in common use today, there are many of us who believe that "Mother" still knows best.

This book is dedicated to the millions of Americans who remember a fond mother (or grandmother) brewing a cup of 'magic' for a sick child; those who recognize that the very bedrock of modern medicine stands on the firm foundation of Mother Nature's Pharmacy.

Preface

Good morning, my friends:

I am sitting here in the thin, hazy sunlight of early morning with my hands on the keys of my battered old Corona portable in front of me, but my thoughts are far away.

I am looking out the window at my own small herb garden, but instead of the green shoots, flowers and fronds of the plants, I see in my mind's eye the shadowy figure of a medieval monk bending between the rows; a kerchiefed woman in a long gown stooping to gather flower heads for the basket on her arm, a child at her heels; a tiny Chinese in brilliantly embroidered robes tenderly digging out gnarled roots; an East Indian gentleman precisely selecting new shoots and leaves; an Egyptian priest consecrating the plants to the Sun God; a Greek physician of the 15th century meticulously drawing and recording the configuration of the plants for posterity; an imposing bearded figure in the constricting clothes of the last century taking cuttings and a native American Indian clad in a loin cloth stashing certain plant parts in a rawhide medicine bag suspended around his neck. I feel quite close to these people somehow, as if I'm part of a continuing and unbroken chain.

The story of the medicinal herbs is as old as recorded history itself. When I began the research for this book so many months ago, I had no idea what fascinating people I would meet along the way or the major contributions the ancient herbologists have made to today's traditional practice of medicine.

Since the advent of chemically synthesized prescription drugs, mankind has neglected the natural medicinal herbs. But even orthodox medical practitioners caution about the harmful side-effects of many of the chemical drugs, and responsible doctors limit their use to a short time period in order to minimize the risks. Although we must all be grateful for the great strides that have been made in modern medicine, it is common knowledge that many drugs are abused.

How much more pleasant it is to drink a cup of herb tea to banish a headache than take two aspirin. Sleep seems more sweet and peaceful when a steaming cup of fragrant herb tea has relaxed every muscle and banished the cares of the day. Herbs allow you to awake refreshed and ready to take on the world without the drug hangover that is the reminder of chemicals that depressed your system the night before.

If you believe, as I do, that the Creator has provided all things for His children, you might want to try His medicinal herbs for the minor aches and pains that plague you. I look forward to a time when our medical doctors not only recognize the contributions of the herbologists of the past, but once again work hand-in-hand with naturalists to employ the healing powers of herbs in conjunction with modern medicine.

Until that happy day arrives, does it not behoove us to gain as much knowledge as we can and use what God gives us to treat our bodies as gently and naturally as possible? But, a word of caution here. The power of herbs is very real and their use is not for the uninitiated. You must not fix up a blend of herbs willy-nilly for tea just because you like the taste of the mixture. Each herb detailed in this book has specific properties and will create a certain action within the body.

Please take the time to become as intimately acquainted with the healing herbs as you would with a treasured friend. Unfortunately, you won't have the benefit of Great-Grandmother looking over your shoulder to slap your hand if you reach for the wrong combination!

With my European heritage, I easily accept the use of the medicinal plants. I still remember my Grandmother consulting the village authority to make certain some of her potions were correct before she administered them. Expertise in the art of herbal healing requires study. But the rewards are great and the knowledge of the healing power of Nature's Pharmacy is very worthwhile.

To your very good health,

William L. Fischer

Chapter 1

...and the fruit thereof shall be for meat,
and the leaf thereof for medicine.
Ezekiel 47:12

THE HISTORY OF HERBOLOGY

Today's medical doctor and the pharmacist he relies upon to dispense the pills and liquids manufactured in giant chemical laboratories owe a lot more to the early hebalists than they might think. In fact, the scientific advances today's pharmacist depends on have their roots in the apothecary shops of yesterday. The modern pharmacist, of course, merely fills prescriptions written by medical doctors. Although most households of the past had their kitchen herb gardens which the chatelaine tended personally, the ancient apothecary meticulously maintained his stock of medicinal herbs and advised his clients on their use as well as standing ready to dispense on the physician's advice.

It was not until the end of the 19th century, the relatively recent past when you consider mankind's long history, that the secrets of preparing synthetic drugs and medicines began to be discovered.

Herbal medicine dates back almost before recorded history. Hundreds of medicinal plants were known and used in India many, many centuries before the Christian era began. As far back as 2735 B.C., the Chinese emperor Shen Nung brushed an authoritative herbal. Herbal medicine thrives in China to this day and the Chinese refer to ancient herbals listing over 1,000 plants, still authoritative and still effective after so many centuries. It is recorded that Egyptian physicians of the 1st and 2nd century A.D. treated constipation with senna pods and used carraway and peppermint to relieve indigestion.

Pliny the Elder and the Greek physician Crateus produced an herbal very early in the 1st century B.C. with hand-colored illustrations of various medicinal plants. This incredible achievement has not survived, but authorities believe the vital information therein was included in the *materia medica* of Pedanius Dioscorides, the master herbalist and famed physician of Greece whose writings testify to the achievements of these early physicians. It is believed that the famed Viennese codex of 512 A.D. is a compilation of the Dioscorides manuscript.

Several herbals were published in medieval Europe around the 15th century, the most famous being Konrad von Megenberg's *Das puch der natur*, sometimes called *Buch der natur* (Book of Nature). Printed in 1475, it included the first known woodcuts of botanical illustrations. In the 1530s, Otto Brunfels' *Herbarium vivae eicones* was published with the excellent and accurate drawings of wood engraver Hans Weiditz. The first real pharmacopeia containing a collection of medicinal chemicals and drugs with specific directions for preparation came from Nuremberg in 1546. Other herbals survive from this period, including a Latin language version of an Aztec manuscript dated around 1552.

In 1617, the Society of Apothecaries was founded in London and only a member of the society could keep an apothecary's shop and make and sell medicinal preparations. In England in 1649, Nicholas Culpepper penned *A Physicall Directory,* a respected pharmacopeia of the time which is still widely referred to and quoted today. By 1841, the Pharmaceutical Society of Great Britain was founded and education and training of these early pharmacists was mandatory.

However, shops with trained apothecaries were only found in the big cities. The published manuscripts were beyond the reach of most persons and herbal lore was traditionally passed from generation to generation by word of mouth. In isolated areas, mother passed her knowledge to daughter; the village "witch" passed his or her knowledge onto some worthy soul with an aptitude and feeling for herbs; early American settlers brought their medicine bags and seeds to the new world so the knowledge and skills would not be lost. These early settlers learned from the Indians of herbs native to this part of the world and the cycle continued.

Today, the orthodox medical establishment looks askance at the herbalist, yet they should not. Medical science owes a great deal to the lowly plants of the fields. For instance, the drug *digitalis,* used as a blood circulation stimulant for heart disease, comes from the common Foxglove (Digitalis purpurea). Foxglove is cultivated on a commercial scale and the extract stabilized and standardized for prescription use only. The Foxglove was used by early herbalists in heart cases where it increases the activity of the heart and arteries. Its most important property is its action in stimulating circulation.

Another case in point is *quinine,* derived from cinchona bark, and used chiefly in the treatment of malaria. For 300 years, quinine was the only effective remedy for malaria. As a treatment for this debilitating disease, quinine has helped more people than any other known drug used to fight any infectious disease. It was not until 1944 that anti-malarial drugs were first synthesized in a laboratory. However, some strains of the malarial parasite developed a resistance to the synthetics in the 1960s and natural quinine was reinstated as the treatment of choice in certain cases.

The opium Poppy (Papaver somniferum) gives us important pain-relieving analgesics and narcotics, such as morphine, codeine and thebaine, plus muscle-relaxers and that age-old treatment for diarrhea, paregoric. Laudanum, a tincture of opium, was a favorite remedy in Victorian days and no medical bag was complete without this early tranquilizer. Even today, morphine, the most important alkaloid of opium, remains the standard against which all new synthetic pain-relievers are measured.

There are probably as many as 800,000 species of plants on this sweet earth. Considering this fact, it is remarkable how few have been cultivated by man as food or medicine. And, with the Biblical injunction ringing in our ears..."and the leaf thereof for medicine," we may be pardoned for wondering what both the ancient herbalists and modern science may have missed.

In our modern times, herbs are available in many forms through herb shops, health food stores and by mail-order purchase from houses specializing in their dissemination.

The most common method of preparing the medicinal herbs for preservation and storage has always been carefully controlled drying. Some current manufacturers of herbal preparations also employ alcohol extraction procedures. These two methods, time-honored and satisfactory, but unfortunately not perfect, both result in a measureable loss of some important active constituents, including enzymes, amino acids and proteins. These procedures also affect the elements vital in stimulating the immune system (such as the large molecular weight polysaccharides), and reduce the properties of the volatile oils and other principles found in the tranquilizing and sedative herbs.

However, thanks to the latest space-age technology, you may now purchase freeze-dried *(lypholized)* botanicals of field-fresh potency. Fresh, freeze-dried and encapsulated botanicals offer therapeutic values never before possible in prepared herbals. Only medicinal herbs prepared and consumed directly from the field exceed the freeze-dried preparations in potency, and then only slightly. In line with the best of naturopathic herbal traditions and current scientific techniques, the pioneers of this costly fresh, freeze-drying technology are able to insure that the biologically active elements of the whole fresh plant are maintained for maximum therapeutic effect.

Fresh freeze-drying captures all the potency and freshness lost in common drying or alcohol-extraction procedures. Not only have chromatographic studies proven that freeze-drying maintains all the vital principles of the fresh botanical, you can verify these results with your own senses. Simply open a capsule and inhale the field-fresh fragrance of the herb. You can even taste the difference in quality! Question your supplier and read labels to determine how capsulized herbals have been processed and do purchase freeze-dried whenever possible. The difference in quality and efficacy more than makes up for the additional cost.

Growing your own herbs is very rewarding and probably many of you will wish to start your own herb garden. If you decide to grow your own, the seed packets you will purchase will give you detailed growing instructions. If you buy young, potted herbs in a nursery, a knowledgeable employee with a green thumb will certainly be glad to pass on his enthusiasm and will instruct you in how to care for your new botanicals. We have given you broad guidelines for each herb as to type of environment each prefers, along with how to harvest, when to harvest, what parts to harvest and how to dry and store the harvested parts. For some reason, this vital information is missing from most sources publishing on herbs.

In addition, with the resurgence of interest in natural medicine and self-care health care, many professional individuals have been trained to teach the proper use of herbs and some offer detailed and involved courses in the use of the traditional medicinal herbs. These courses are fascinating, informative, inexpensive and fun.

In the following pages, you will find a compendium of many of the most important medicinal herbs, along with their history and current and past usage. This book is as complete as research will allow. We have endeavored to provide the most authoritative modern text currently in publication on Nature's Pharmacy.

Chapter 2
HARVESTING, DRYING, PREPARING & STORING HERBS GENERAL DIRECTIONS

Although each chapter gives specific information on growing, harvesting, drying, preparing and storing the particular herb being discussed, the following general guidelines pertain to all herbs and will insure your success in the gentle art of herbology.

HARVESTING: Whether you are harvesting herbs for immediate use in the fresh state or for drying, they should be gathered at the time during their growing cycle when they are most potent. Flowers are at their strongest during the beginning of flowering. Leaves are most vigorous just before the buds open, but also may be taken during the time of flowering. Fruits are harvested as they become ripe. Roots should be dug out only when the plant is in a dormant phase, either early spring or late fall. It is best to gather the medicinal plants no earlier than mid-morning on a sunny day. There are two reasons for this. First, the sun must have had time to dry the moisture which has accumulated overnight in the form of dew. Second, the plants which are heated by a hot sun are at their most potent state because the volatile oils are free-flowing and strongest when the plants are warmed. As a general rule of thumb, it is best to schedule your harvesting time from around 10:00 AM until around 3:00 PM.

You will, of course, select only clean, healthy plants which show no insect infestation in the form of chewed leaves, mites on the underside of leaves, or ragged blossoms. If you are gathering in the field instead of your own garden, bypass roadsides and highways where the plants will have been contaminated by traffic. Herbs growing near railway embankments, dirty streams or industrial plants are also unsuitable for harvesting. Fields, meadows, woodlands and pastures are usually excellent sources of herbs in the wild, but watch out for grazing land which may have been chemically fertilized by a neighboring farmer anxious to provide good grasses for his animals.

Please be as considerate when field-gathering as you would be when harvesting in your own garden. Don't pull plants out by their roots and don't leave a mess behind you. Always leave several plants of a given species to insure sufficient growth for future harvests. When gathering leaves and blossoms only, snick them off between your fingernails and you will do minimum damage to the plant. Pinching is preferable to cutting because the pinch acts to close the broken stem and helps seal in the plant's vital juices. You may, when necessary, scissor tough stems when gathering the entire herb, but leave at least one growing stem so the plant can heal itself. If you are gathering roots, please dig them out carefully and, when possible, divide the root clump and replant a portion of it to insure future growth.

The time-honored method of carrying herbs home is to layer them loosely in an open basket. There's a reason for this. You must take care not to crush delicate blossoms and leaves. If the leaves and blossoms are crushed and the stems broken, some of the vital oils can escape, reducing the herb's medicinal properties.

If you don't have a basket handy, use a brown paper bag. But don't ever carry home your prizes in plastic. Harmful condensation will form as the plants sweat inside the plastic. You may not even notice that any damage has been done until the drying process has been completed and the herbs turn black, rendering them useless as medicinals.

DRYING: Herbs selected for drying should not be washed. When drying the entire plant, tie several stems together loosely and hang the bunch upside down in a warm, airy place until thoroughly dry. When drying leaves or flowers, they must be spread out without touching each other in a single layer on a white cloth or unprinted paper. Butcher paper, shelf lining paper (if not printed or glazed), and brown-paper bags opened up and pressed flat are all suitable. A finely-meshed screen which allows air to circulate all around the herb parts is best of all.

Roots, barks or thick, fleshy herb parts may be dried in a very slow oven (no higher than 100 degrees F.) to hasten the process. If you have a gas oven, often the pilot light alone will provide sufficient heat. Roots should be scrubbed clean and cut into smaller segments to insure thorough drying. Mistletoe and the Small-Flowered Willow Herbs may also be cut before drying, but do not wash.

You may do your drying outdoors, but not in direct sunlight. The only drawback to using summer's hot temperatures to accomplish the drying process is that the herbs must be brought indoors overnight so as not to gather moisture. Any warm, well-ventilated room provides a suitable atmosphere for drying herbs. An attic is first choice, but a spare room or unused bedroom will do. The kitchen is not a good choice because cooking odors can permeate the herbs and the laundry is not suitable because it is usually full of steamy, moisture-laden air.

Before storing dried herbs, test to make sure they are thoroughly dry. Fully dried parts will break or powder when broken with the fingers. Store your dried herbs in glass jars or small boxes which can be made air-tight. Green or amber jars which protect your precious herbs from light are best. Keep the containers in a dark, dry cupboard and the medicinal properties will remain volatile through the winter.

There are two 'don'ts' when storing herbs. Don't use plastic or metal containers, and don't be greedy. You can't store vast quantities and expect them to last for years. Dried herbs lose quality as time passes and should be used within six to eight months for best results. Fortunately, Nature's Pharmacy is self-renewing and a new supply of herbs will thrust up their green shoots every spring, as they have done since time began.

METHODS OF PREPARATION: Specific instructions for preparing each herb are detailed in the text of the various chapters, including the length of time required for steeping the particular herb as an infusion, but some general guidelines are useful as well.

HOW TO PREPARE A HOT INFUSION (TEA): Fresh or dried herbs in suitable quantity (see individual chapters) are measured and placed in a china or glass teapot or cup. Plastic and metal containers are not suitable for steeping herbs. For each cup, 6 ounces of freshly boiled water is poured over the herbs. Cover and steep as directed in the individual chapters. As a general rule, fresh herbs are steeped from 30 to 60 seconds while dried herbs are steeped from two to four minutes. The resulting tea should be light in color and delicate to the taste.

If a steeped infusion is to be taken throughout the day, prepare the entire quantity at one time and place it in a thermos to keep it at a comfortable sipping temperature.

When preparing a hot infusion from a root, chop the root coarsely and place it in a suitable amount of cold water. Bring the mixture to a boil and steep, covered, for three minutes. When a root infusion is recommended, the individual chapters will give further detail.

HOW TO PREPARE A COLD INFUSION (TEA): Certain herbs, such as Calamus, Mallow and Mistletoe, lose considerable medicinal properties when heat is applied. A tea from these herbs is made with a cold infusion. To prepare a cold infusion, measure out a suitable quantity of the herb, and soak overnight in cold water. The following morning, you may warm slightly to sipping temperature, strain, and store your daily ration in a thermos. To maintain warmth, rinse the thermos in hot water before adding the tea.

HOW TO MIX COLD & HOT INFUSIONS: Because some elements are released by heat and some leached out by soaking in cold water, a blending of both hot and cold infusions insures full medicinal properties. Soak the recommended amount of the herb in just half the amount of cold water specified in the individual chapters. The following morning, strain off the liquid and retain the residue. Bring the other half of the specified amount of water to a boil and pour over the residue. Allow the mixture to steep, covered, for a few minutes and then combine the hot infusions with the cold. In this way, the active elements released by both heat and cold are obtained.

HOW TO PREPARE A TINCTURE (ESSENCE): Loosely fill a glass bottle with the fresh or dried herbs and add pure spirits, such as vodka, to cover. Cork tightly and allow to stand in a warm place (approximately 70 degrees F.) for at least two weeks. Shake the mixture daily during the waiting period. After the two weeks have passed, strain and squeeze out the residue. Tinctures are commonly given as drops in herb tea or diluted in a little water. They may also be employed as a compress or in a massage. See individual chapters for details of specific use.

HOW TO PREPARE AN HERBAL OIL: Flowers or herb parts, as specified in the individual chapters, should be placed loosely in a glass (not plastic) bottle. Slowly add cold-pressed, unrefined olive oil until the oil level is an inch above the herb parts. Cork tightly and allow the bottle to stand in a very warm place for two weeks. You may place the oil near the stove to gather warmth from cooking or outside in the hot sun. Just remember to bring it in before night cools the air.

HOW TO PREPARE AN OINTMENT: The certain herbs which are suitable for use in an ointment are detailed in the individual chapters. An ointment is prepared by heating 2 cups of pure lard (not vegetable shortening) to a temperature suitable for making french fries. Add four big handfuls of finely chopped herbs (scissors make it easy) to the hot fat and stir to blend. The herb parts will sizzle and crackle, so beware of splattering fat. After 60 seconds, remove from heat and cover. Allow the blend to stand overnight. The following morning, heat gently to liquify and squeeze through cheesecloth to remove the residue. Place the filtered ointment in glass jars and store as directed in the individual chapters.

Note: Before passing through the cheesecloth, you may wish to add 4 tablespoons of cold-pressed, unrefined olive oil to ointments which must be stored under refrigeration to help keep them from completely solidifying in the cold. Because an icy-cold ointment is unpleasant to use, you may wish to employ a hot-water bath to warm up the mixture before applying it. Put the jar in a container and add very hot water to the container until the water is nearly up to the jar lid. Allow the ointment to remain in the hot water bath until it has warmed to a comfortable temperature.

HOW TO PREPARE FRESH JUICE: Wash the herbs well under cold running water and place them still wet in the juice extractor. If necessary, scissor into pieces of a suitable size. These fresh juices are often used internally in the form of drops diluted in tea or water. The fresh juice may also be recommended for dabbing on certain affected parts of the body. See individual chapters for recommended use. Note: Fresh juices are generally used immediately after extraction. However, you may place the drops in a small bottle, cork tightly, and hold refrigerated for several days without an appreciable loss of the vital properties.

HOW TO PREPARE A STEAMED POULTICE OR COMPRESS: Place a colander, strainer or sieve over a pot containing rapidly boiling water. Layer either fresh or dried herbs in the colander, reduce heat to simmering temperature, cover, and allow the steam to wilt and penetrate the herbal parts. After about five minutes, put the soft, warm herbs into a clean, white, loosely-woven cloth envelope and apply to the affected area. Overwrap in a woolen cloth to hold in the heat. The poultice should remain in place for at least two hours and may be left on overnight.

HOW TO PREPARE A PULP POULTICE OR COMPRESS: Place a quantity of fresh herb parts on a clean white cloth and crush to a pulp with a rolling pin. Apply to the affected area of the body and bandage well with a woolen overwrap. A pulp poultice can remain in place overnight.
Note: Crushing the herbs directly onto a cloth retains all juices, which improves the efficiency of the compress.

HOW TO PREPARE A FULL BATH, A SITZ BATH OR A WASH: The method of preparation for a full bath, a sitz bath or a wash is the same; only the quantities differ. As recommended in the individual chapters for a particular use, a measured amount of the herb is soaked in cold water overnight. The following morning, the mixture is heated and strained and a suitable quantity is added to the water for a full bath, sitz bath or wash.

For a full bath, approximately 7 ounces of dried herbs or 6 quarts of fresh herbal parts are used. After the infusion is warmed and added to the bath, enjoy a good twenty minute soak while making sure the heart region remains above the water level. Upon leaving the bath, do not take time to dry. Immediately wrap up in a robe or outsize bath towel, go to bed, and cover up warmly to induce perspiration. Relax for an hour.

For a sitz bath, approximately 3 ounces of dried herbs or 2-1/2 quarts of fresh herbal parts are used. Warm the infusion and add to the sitz bath. In this instance, the water must cover the area of the kidneys.

For an herbal wash, approximately 1 ounce of dried herbs or 2 cups of the fresh herbal parts are used.

Note: These infused waters may be rewarmed and used three times in all before they lose their potency. Individual chapters give detailed instruction on preparation and use of the various herbs recommended for baths and washes.

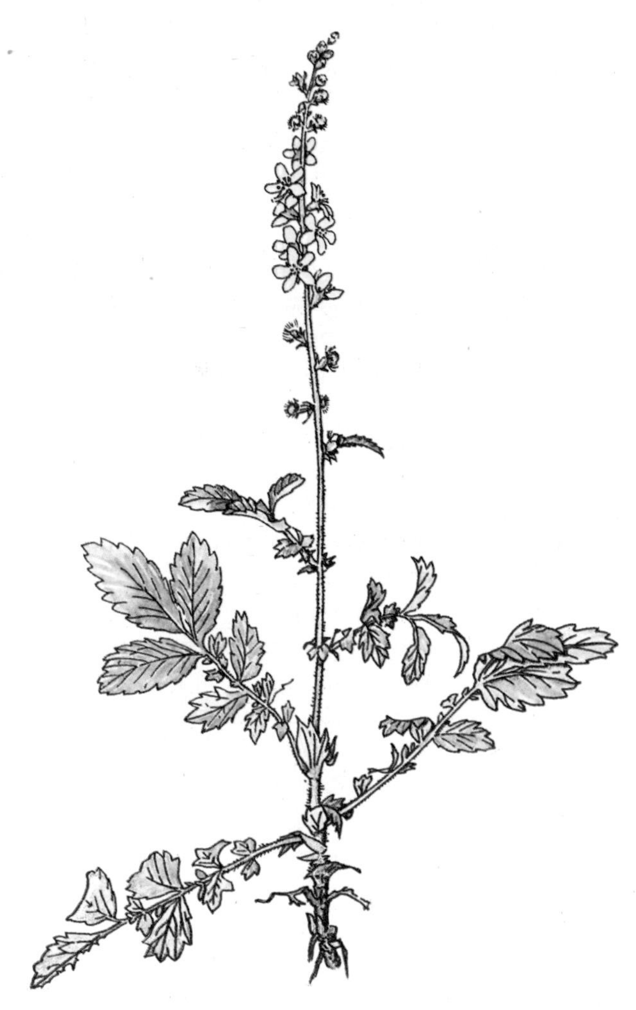

Agrimony

Agrimonia eupatoria

Chapter 3
AGRIMONY
(Agrimonia eupatoria)

Anemia
Bladder Disorders
Bladder Infections
Digestive Problems
Heart (enlarged)
Kidneys
Liver
Lumbago
Lungs
Mouth (inflamed)
Rheumatism
Sores (scrofulous)
Skin
Spleen Disorders
Stomach Complaints
Throat Disorders
Tonsillitis
Varicose Veins
Wounds

PAST HISTORY: Ancient Egyptian healers put this herb to good use, and, by the Middle Ages, magic powers were attributed to 'Egrimoyne.' An old English pharmacopeia had this to say: *'If it be leyd under mann's heed, He shal sleepyn as he were deed; He shal never drede ne wakyn, Till fro under his heed it be takyn.'* Although Agrimony is not a narcotic, it was believed to induce a heavy dreamless sleep which allowed the ingestor to awaken refreshed.

Agrimony was often mixed with Mugwort and vinegar for a bad back and all open wounds. At least one old herbalist recommended a rather questionable blend of Agrimony, pounded frogs and human blood as a cure for internal bleeding.

The botanical name for this plant comes from the Greek 'Argemone' and Mithridates Eupator, a Greek ruler famous for his herbal remedies. Agrimony once held an honored place in the *Materia Medica* of the London Pharmacopeia Society, was recommended for 'naughty livers' and is still very much appreciated by herbalists today.

DESCRIPTION & GROWING REQUIREMENTS: Agrimony has small yellow flowers clustered together on graceful slender spiky stems and often attains a height of three feet. The entire plant is covered with a downy hair and the large leaves grow near the ground.

Agrimony prefers a sunny, dry location, will tolerate light shade and is often found wild on the edges of fields and woods. It is easily started from seed and thrives in rock gardens or as a border plant.

HOW TO HARVEST & STORE: The leaves are harvested from June to August when the plant is in full flower. Gather the complete plant and dry the flowers and leaves by tying small bunches together and hanging whole stalks upside down in a dry airy place.

LEGENDARY CURES: Agrimony was the prime ingredient of the famed 'arquebusade water' used to heal wounds inflicted by an arquebus (hand gun) in the 13th century.

The diary of Philip de Comines described the horrors of the battle of Morat in 1476 and praised the healing of arquebusade water. Eau de arquebusade water is still widely used in France today with notable success for sprains and bruises.

TRADITIONAL USE — INTERNALLY: Agrimony leaf tea offers great healing qualities for throat and mouth inflammation, tonsillitis and all types of throat disorders. Many lecturers and singers use Agrimony tea as a gargle to clear their voices.

The beneficial astringency of Agrimony makes it especially valuable in problems of the liver. Kidney and bladder infections have been known to yield to Agrimony.

A noted European herbalist recommends 2 cups of Agrimony tea daily for anemia, wounds, rheumatism, lumbago, long-standing digestive difficulties, liver and spleen disorders. Up to 3 cups daily constitutes a powerful remedy for enlargement of the heart, stomach trouble, lungs, kidney and bladder disorders.

TRADITIONAL USE — EXTERNALLY: The ointment is especially helpful in relieving varicose veins and sores on the lower limbs. A healing bath of Agrimony once or twice a year soothes the skin. Children suffering with scrofulous sores which are hard to heal will benefit with a daily bath.

PREPARING AGRIMONY TEA: Pour 1 pint of boiling water over 1 teaspoon of fresh or dried Agrimony. Cover closely and allow to steep for 5 minutes.

PREPARING AN AGRIMONY BATH: Steep two handfuls of fresh or dried Agrimony overnight in approximately 6 quarts of fresh cold water. The following morning, heat, strain, and add the liquid to a full bath.

AGRIMONY INFUSION (TEA) FOR LIVER DISORDERS: Mix equal parts of Agrimony, Cleavers (see Chapter 8) and Woodruff. Add 1 heaping teaspoon of the blend to 1 cup boiling water. Cover and allow to steep for 5 minutes.

PREPARING AGRIMONY OINTMENT: Gently heat 2 cups pure lard (not vegetable shortening) just until it begins to bubble. Blend 2 handfuls of finely chopped leaves, stems and flowers and add. Cover the mixture and allow to cool overnight. The next day, warm to liquify and strain through cheesecloth, using the hands to press out the residue of the herbs. Pour into clean jars and refrigerate. Use a hot-water bath to warm before use.
Note: A tablespoon or two of cold-pressed olive oil may be added to help keep the blend pliable under refrigeration.

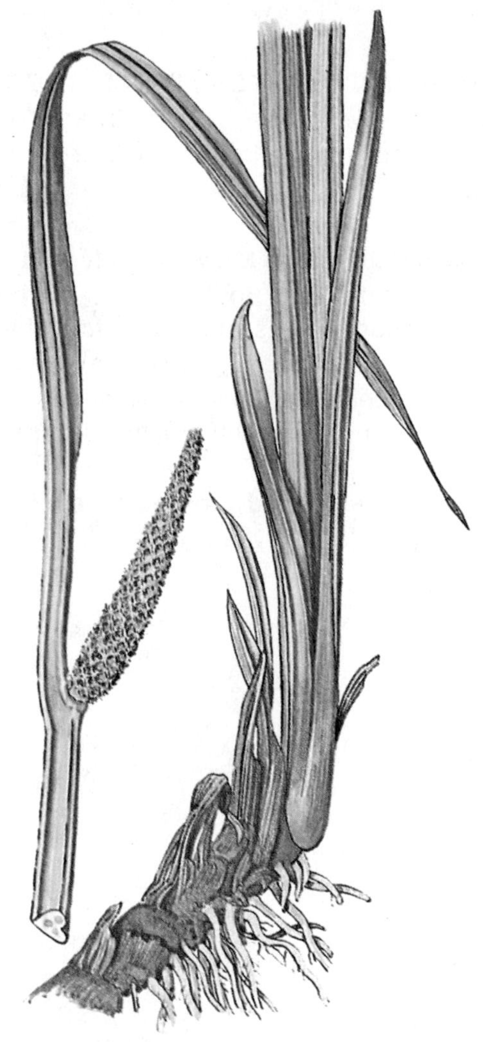

Calamus — Sweet Flag

Acorus calamus

Chapter 4
CALAMUS — SWEET FLAG
(Acorus calamus)

Appetite	*Eyes (weak/tired)*	*Kidneys*
Cancer (lungs)	*Flatulence*	*Liver*
Cancer (intestines)	*Frostbite*	*Metabolism (faulty)*
Colic	*Gall Bladder*	*Pancreas*
Chilblains	*Gastro-Intestinal Tract*	*Smokers Aid*
Diarrhea (bloody)	*Glandular Disorders*	*Spleen*
*Digestive Disorders**	*Gout*	*Stomach Pains*
		Ulcers (duodenal)

**Including difficulty digesting wheat and grain products.*

PAST HISTORY: The sweet, spicy, and lemony scent of Calamus made it a favorite in medieval times as a strewing herb. Calamus was gathered and scattered on damp, cold stone floors where its strong odor was released when crushed underfoot.

Pieces of the root were often dried and used as sachets to perfume clothing chests and cupboards where its fragrance served to hide the fact that people bathed just once a year, if then. The common folk, who could not afford expensive imported flavorings like cinnamon, ginger and nutmeg, often used Calamus as a spicy addition in cooking.

Internally, Calamus root was dried and powdered and used as an infusion for fevers and dyspepsia. Pieces of the dried root were chewed in small bits as a digestive aid and to clear hoarseness of the throat.

DESCRIPTION & GROWING REQUIREMENTS: Like the common cattail it resembles, Calamus is a water-loving plant and grows wild in marshes and on the banks of ponds and lakes. It develops strong leaves shaped like a sword which grow from a sheath at the base. The "flower" stalk projects at almost a right angle from the axils of its outer leaves.

You may grow Calamus easily at home as long as you are prepared to satisfy its tremendous thirst by giving it abundant water. Divide the root clumps in early spring or autumn, set the baby plants about twelve

inches apart, cover them well and water them often.
Note: Calamus flowers only when grown in water.

HOW TO HARVEST & STORE: The roots should be harvested in very early spring or late autumn when the plant is resting. It is best to give the plant two years growth before harvesting or dividing the roots to allow it to fully develop before interrupting growth. Dry the roots and store whole, chopped or even powdered. Be sure to peel the root before chopping or powdering.

Dry the leaves and roots by putting them in a single layer, preferably on a screen so air can circulate around them. They will dry nicely outside during the hot summer months, but must be kept out of the direct sun. Cover them lightly against insects.

LEGENDARY CURES: A startling cure which Calamus accomplished is the case of a middle-aged man, Norman E., who was dying of cancer of the lungs. He was mere skin and bones and his physician had given him up as terminal when he was advised by a friend to chew Calamus root and to drink Yarrow tea (see Chapter 33) every morning and evening. Mr. E. decided he had nothing to lose and everything to gain. He followed his friend's advice to the letter and slowly began to gain weight and felt better and better as time went on. After about six months of this self-treatment, Norman E. returned to his doctor who confessed he thought his patient had died! You can imagine the doctor's surprise upon finding the patient had cured himself with simple herbs. I would like to be able to tell you this able physician now prescribes Calamus root and Yarrow tea, but I suspect he continues to scoff at such old-fashioned remedies.

One of the most celebrated herbalists in Europe first became interested in natural medicine after Calamus root healed her beloved mother of intestinal cancer. The older woman was suffering from excruciating abdominal pains, had lost a tremendous amount of weight and was very weak when her daughter heard a natural physician speaking of Calamus root on a radio broadcast. The doctor said every disorder of the stomach and intestines, whether it was new, old or even malignant, could be healed by taking one sip of a Calamus root infusion (tea) before and after each of the three daily meals. He directed one level teaspoon of Calamus root (powdered and dried) be soaked overnight in a cup of cold water. After warming the tea in a waterbath the following day, the total of six sips per day is taken.

The loving daughter prepared this miraculous healing tea and persuaded her skeptical mother to take it as directed. After only two weeks, the patient was free of pain and began to gain much-needed weight. This renowned herbalist says Calamus root has given the same healing relief in many cases known to her personally. This folk remedy benefits the entire gastro-intestinal tract, plus the liver, gall bladder, spleen and pancreas.

Many more inspiring stories of the benefits of the Calamus root have come to us from Europe. Mind you, these are recent reports, not legends from the historical past.

For instance, a man, Roy W., in his mid-forties suffering from a serious case of bloody diarrhea for over ten years was understandably so weak he was unable to work and care for his family. After taking six sips of Calamus root tea daily along with two cups of Calendula tea (see Chapter 5) for two months, Mr. W.'s condition improved so rapidly he was once again able to work.

Shirley B. was on medication for many years for a duodenal ulcer, could not tolerate solid foods and had completely lost her appetite for even the most dainty tidbits. Mrs. B. lived daily with pain and suffering. After trying Calamus root tea in the recommended six daily sips for a little over a month, she found her appetite again and was able to enjoy a meal with her family for the first time in many, many months.

Another woman, Mary M., taking strong medication daily for undiagnosed stomach pains, discovered Calamus root tea and found the pain was conquered after only three days and has not returned.

TRADITIONAL USE — INTERNALLY: As you can see, Calamus root is an exceptionally potent and powerful herb beneficial in many instances of ill health. It is in widespread use today in Europe and is noted for strengthening the digestive system by stimulating the stomach juices, intestinal tract and kidneys. It overcomes flatulence and colic and is helpful in treating glandular disorders and gout.

Calamus improves the appetite, being especially useful in convalescence or weight loss caused by a faulty metabolism. As a cleansing agent for the entire body, it has no equal in herbal lore. A weak tea can be given to children who have difficulty in digesting wheat and grain products. Of special interest to many, it should be noted that chewing a bit of dried Calamus root is a tremendous aid to smokers who have tried (and perhaps failed many times) to break the habit.

Although the taste of the fresh herb is bitter and pungent, the dried root is relatively mild and might just be the miracle cure that gets the monkey off the smoker's back once and for all.

TRADITIONAL USE – EXTERNALLY: Tired and weakened eyes can be strengthened by dabbing a cotton pad soaked with the freshly pressed juice of a Calamus root over the eyelid. Allow the juice to remain for a few moments before rinsing off thoroughly with cool water.

Even today, in the mountainous regions of Europe where chilblains and frostbite are common, an infusion or full bath of Calamus, slightly warmed, is used to relieve the almost unbearable pain of thawing extremities. The afflicted parts are simply immersed in the bath for twenty minutes at a time. The same mixture can be used up to four times before it loses its potency.

PREPARING CALAMUS TEA: Soak one teaspoon of Calamus root in a pint of cold water overnight. Warm slightly in the morning and strain off the residue. Before using, warm the tea in a waterbath.
Note: Calamus root tea should be prepared only as a cold infusion as directed above. Do not steep this herb in boiling water.

PREPARING FRESH CALAMUS ROOT JUICE: Clean the fresh roots thoroughly, scrubbing off all clinging soil. While the roots are still wet, put them through a juice extractor.

PREPARING A FULL CALAMUS BATH: Soak about 8 ounces of Calamus roots in 5 quarts of cold water overnight. The following day, bring this infusion to a boil, strain, and add to the bath water.

Chapter 5
CALENDULA — MARIGOLD
(Calendula officinalis)

Athlete's Foot
Bedsores
Blood Purifier
Bruises
Burns
Cancer (skin)
Circulatory System
Contusions
Diarrhea (chronic)
Feet (dry/cracked)
Fistulas
Frostbite
Fungal Infections
Intestinal Disorders
Genitals
Glandular Swellings
Hepatitis
Liver Disorders
Liver-spots
Mastectomy (post)
Phlebitis
Scabies
Skin Conditions
Skin Ulcers
Sores (festering)
Sprains/Swellings
Stomach Cramps
Strawberry-Marks
Typhus
Ulcers
Viral Infections
Urine (infected)
Warts
Wounds
Varicose Veins

PAST HISTORY: Calendula, better known as the Marigold, was a kitchen garden staple in medieval times and is a well-known ornamental plant as well as a powerful herb. Marigold flowers were used to give cheese (and hair) a bright yellow color and no broth was considered 'well made' by a good cook without the addition of dried Marigolds.

The *Maison Rustique*, often called "The Countrie Farme," which was penned in 1699, named Marigold as a specific for headaches, jaundice, red eyes, toothaches and ague, and says, "A conserve made of the flowers and sugar taken in the morning fasting, cureth the trembling of the harte and is also given in times of plague or pestilence."

The Marigold was so popular in early 15th century Europe that apothecaries and the spice sellers shops of the time had barrels filled with dried Marigolds for purchase. Master Herbalist Culpepper said, "The flowers, either green or dried, are much used in possets, broths and drinks, as a comforter of the heart and spirits and to expel any malignant or pestilential quality which might annoy."

As much superstition as fact surrounds the early use of Marigolds. One old herbalist wrote, "It must be taken only when the moon is in the Sign of the Virgin and not when Jupiter is in ascendant. The gatherer,

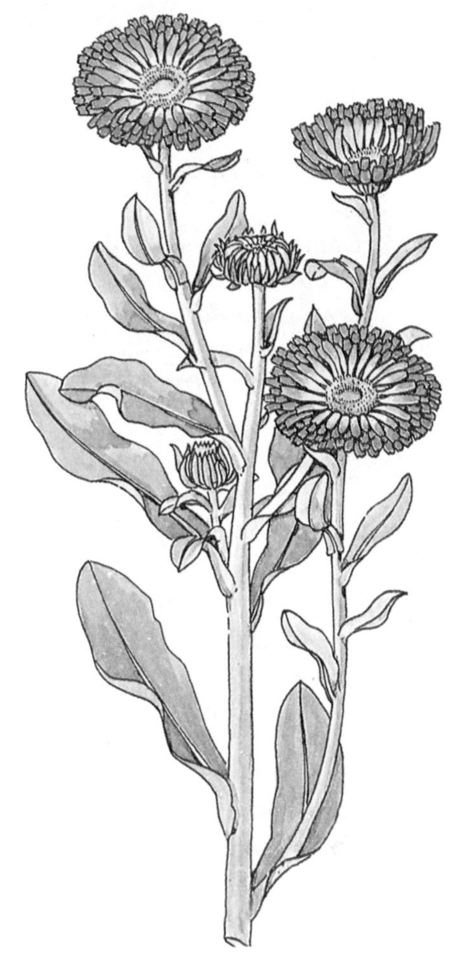

Calendula — Marigold

Calendula officinalis

who must be out of deadly sin, must say three Pater Nosters and three Aves. It will then give the wearer a vision of anyone who has robbed him." Another old wive's tale says when the flowers close after 7 o'clock in the morning, it will rain the same day.

DESCRIPTION & GROWING REQUIREMENTS: The colorful and familiar yellow-orange flowers of the Marigold make a bright spot in the garden and Marigold is a superior bedding plant. The stems and leaves of the Marigold are thick and somewhat sticky and the plant is exceedingly easy to grow from seed. Sow the seeds thinly in early spring in just about any type of soil.

The Marigold likes full sun, but will tolerate a partially shady location just as well. When the plants are young, thin them out to about ten inches apart, keep the bed free of weeds, and stand back! Marigolds reseed themselves and will spread out as far as you let them if allowed to grow as they wish.

HOW TO HARVEST & STORE: Gather the flower heads in quantity as they appear and spread out loosely on a screen, but do not allow them to touch or they will discolor. Put them in a warm airy place to dry. A few of the dried flowers added to the soup pot will reward you with a rich golden broth and make a particularly nice addition to chicken soup.

Harvest the leaves and stems in the morning after the sun has dried the dew. Both the flowers and leaves should be gathered in the full sun when the medicinal qualities of the plant are heightened. You may also gather the entire stalk, tie into small bundles and hang upside down in a warm airy place until the entire plant is dry.

LEGENDARY CURES: There are so many stories surrounding the potency and power of Calendula that it's difficult to choose ones most indicative of the benefits of this herb. For instance, little Susie H., less than three years old, required repeated hospitalizations for treatment of the dreaded typhus. She suffered from chronic diarrhea, had lost a great deal of weight and wasn't able to digest sufficient food to support her frail body. The doctors feared for her very life.

Once her mother started her on Calendula tea sweetened with honey, the diarrhea disappeared and the child was once again able to eat. After three weeks, clinical tests showed no further evidence of the typhoid bacillus. A neighbor of mine told me not long ago that Calendula tea cleared up long-standing diarrhea for her after Chamomile tea and the doctor's administrations had both failed.

In another amazing instance, Calendula tea apparently healed a medical doctor of inflammation of the large intestine, a condition he had suffered with for over five years. Dr. H. G. took 2 cups of Calendula tea daily for a week and, although he started out by laughing at the idea of a modern medical man treating himself with herbs, he ended up being both surprised and grateful. I understand Dr. G. has since recommended this method to several patients.

But the most incredible successes of all must be attributed to external applications of Calendula ointment and tinctures. Even as the herbalists of old used Calendula against skin cancer and fungus, so the modern herbalist and naturopaths do also. Calendula ointment was used successfully to hasten the healing of a huge mastectomy wound in a woman whose breast had to be removed. Indeed, her healing was so remarkable compared to other patients, that only a short term radium treatment was used.

In her later years, my own mother suffered dreadfully from varicose veins that pained her constantly. Grandmother was horrified when she noted this condition after we had not seen each other for a long while. She spread Calendula ointment about 1/8th inch thick on mother's legs and wrapped them loosely with clean strips of cloth. By the time we left Grandmother's farm after a month-long visit, the varicose veins had receded and Mother's legs no longer ached. Mother took several jars of the ointment home with her and was able to help two of her friends who also had varicose veins.

A practicing herbologist reports that Calendula ointment can cure the most stubborn case of athlete's foot. This common fungus infection causes unbearable itching and burning. Very often, whole areas of the foot break open and supperate. This herbologist tells of a particularly bad case that would not respond to any form of treatment. The poor man hated to wear anything on his feet at all because his socks would stick to the open sores, causing agony when they had to be removed. After just a week using Calendula ointment, the open sores healed and the terrible itching was relieved.

TRADITIONAL USE — INTERNALLY: Although most American medical doctors do not believe in herbal treatment, many European medical men make use of their powers with great success. Along with many herbalists abroad, I can name at least four or five renowned doctors who strongly recommend Calendula tea in cancer cases. Even when it is known an operation cannot help, they say Calendula tea should be taken daily for a long period. The tea cleanses the blood and stimulates circulation as well.

Calendula tea is beneficial for gastro-intestinal disorders, stomach cramps and ulcers, quiets inflammation of the intestines and is considered excellent against hard-to-treat virus infections and blood and bacteria in the urine. In cases of infectious hepatitis and all disorders of the liver, Calendula tea is suggested for its blood cleansing properties. For any liver involvement, the flowers, leaves and stems should be brewed with boiling water and 3 or 4 cups should be taken daily a tablespoon at a time every 15 minutes. Do not sweeten this mixture.

TRADITIONAL USE — EXTERNALLY: Calendula ointment offers relief of wounds, varicose veins, phlebitis, fistulas, frostbite, burns of all kinds and fungus infections. The fresh juice of Calendula helps heal rough cancer-like skin conditions and has been known to fade strawberry-marks and 'liver spots' (those brown freckle-like spots which come with age), when the areas affected are covered with the fresh juice several times a day over a long period. This ointment even quickly heals scabs inside the nostrils.

The fresh pressed juice also gets rid of warts and scabies and a boiled infusion is said to heal lesions and glandular swellings when the affected areas are bathed in it. Dry cracked feet, open skin ulcers and wounds which refuse to heal are relieved by bathing with Calendula. If the genitals develop a fungus infection, a sitz bath can give relief.

Calendular tincture, diluted with boiling water and used as a compress, relieves wounds, contusions, bruises and sprains and helps heal festering open sores, bedsores and swellings.

PREPARING CALENDULA TEA: Pour a pint of boiling water over 2 heaping teaspoons of fresh Calendula parts (or 1 teaspoon dried), cover and allow to steep for a few minutes. Strain and sip as needed.

PREPARING FRESH JUICE: Gather a quantity of fresh flowers, stems and leaves. Wash gently in cold running water. While still wet, put through a juice extractor.

PREPARING A SITZ BATH: Steep two handfuls fresh Calendula parts (or one handful dried) in a quantity of cold water overnight. Next morning, heat gently, strain, and add to your sitz bath.

PREPARING A WASH: Use 2 heaping tablespoons fresh (or 1 heaping tablespoon dried) Calendula parts to a pint of cold water and proceed as above.

PREPARING A TINCTURE: Fill a glass bottle loosely with fresh Calendula flowers, leaves and stems and cover with alcohol or fruit spirits. (Do not use rubbing alcohol.) Cover tightly and keep the bottle in a warm place (about 70 to 75 degrees F.) for two weeks before use.

PREPARING AN OINTMENT: Gather about two handfuls of fresh Calendula flowers, stems and leaves and chop finely. On low heat, liquify 2 cups of pure lard (not vegetable shortening), add the minced herb and stir. Remove from heat, cover and allow the mixture to stand overnight. Warm gently the next day and strain through cheesecloth, pressing with your hands. You may add a few tablespoons of cold pressed olive oil if you wish to help keep the mass smooth. Pour into clean jars and refrigerate.

Chapter 6
CARROT (Daucus carota)

Arthritis
Diabetes
Digestive Tract
Diuretic
Cancer
Catarrh
Eyes
Gastric Disturbances
Glandular Systems
Gout
Hair Loss (premature)
Immune System
Infections
Intestines
Kidneys
Liver Complaints
Nervous System
Night-Blindness
Respiratory System
Rheumatism
Sinuses
Skin Conditions
Sterility
Throat
Tonsils
Ulcers
Vision
Vigor (restores)
Wounds (supperating)

PAST HISTORY: The carrot is most likely a native wild plant of the coastal regions of southern Europe and was widely cultivated by many ancient civilizations. Writing about the medicinal value of the plant, Pliny says: "The cultivated has the same virtues as the wild variety, although the latter is more powerful, especially when growing in stony places."

Old herbals recommend the use of the seeds as well as the root. According to these writings, the seeds are very useful against gas, colic, hiccoughs, dysentery and chronic coughs. Carrot tea was considered a particularly valuable remedy for chronic kidney diseases, afflictions of the bladder and in the treatment of dropsy.

The name 'Carrot' comes from the Celtic and means 'red of color.' Its botannical name, 'Daucus,' is from the Greek *dias,* meaning 'to burn' and is representative of the carrot's stimulating qualities. One of the oldest surviving mentions of the carrot is in a Greek cookbook written in 230 A.D.

The carrot was first introduced to England during the reign of Queen Elizabeth I by refugees fleeing from the persecutions of Philip II of Spain, as was its cousin, the parsnip. The carrot was immediately welcomed by the British peasantry and gentry alike. In the time of James I, aristocratic ladies of fashion used the feathery leaves as decoration in their elaborate hair-dresses. There is evidence that the carrot was grown in the U.S. in the Virginia colony as early as 1609.

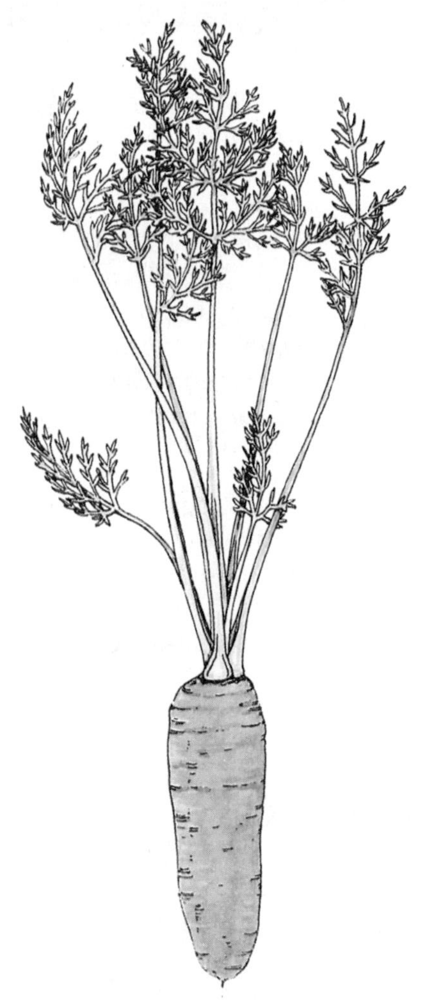

Carrot

Daucus carota

DESCRIPTION & GROWING REQUIREMENTS: This familiar vegetable probably needs no introduction. Those who do not grow it have undoubtedly brought home the fresh variety from farmer's roadside stands or their grocery. In preparing your garden for carrots, it is necessary to provide a deeply cultivated bed of well-fertilized light soil in a sunny location. You will need to dig down at least a foot and spade in some sand or vermiculite to make sure the soil remains loose in order to give the roots easy growing space. Otherwise, the vegetable will be stunted and you will harvest stubby hard roots for your table.

HOW TO HARVEST & STORE: As your crop reaches maturity, probably in the early fall, the easiest method of harvest is to dig them out gently with a pitchfork. If you wish to store them fresh, bury the roots in a box of fine sand and keep the box in a dark, dry place for future use. Your carrots should remain usable until the following spring.

LEGENDARY CURES: With its abundant Vitamin A (alpha and beta carotene), often called 'the eye vitamin,' the carrot is one of the very best aids for strengthening poor vision. The story of Elizabeth K., a young mother of two, very clearly illustrates what the lowly carrot can do in the case of night-blindness arising as a consequence of a deficiency of Vitamin A.

This young woman arranged her life so that she would never have to drive at night. Her night-blindness was very severe and she feared being behind the wheel from dusk on, recognizing her inability to see clearly under these conditions. But, as luck would have it, her husband was off on a business trip when one of the children went into convulsions. The young mother was terrified and bundled both little ones into the car and started off for the hospital at 15 miles per hour. She arrived without incident and the child was successfully treated. But Elizabeth realized that she must do something about her night-blindness because, in an emergency, she might be forced to drive at night and the next time might not be so fortunate.

The following day, Elizabeth bought a juicer and began juicing and drinking a full quart of fresh carrot juice every day. Her husband joked she was 'turning yellow,' but she persisted and even served each member of the family a glass of carrot juice at breakfast. After only a few weeks, Elizabeth found her night-blindness was clearing. She continued on her self-imposed regimen and now drives at night with complete confidence.

TRADITIONAL USE - INTERNALLY: Carrots provide an ample supply of Vitamins A, B, C, D, E, G and K. They are appreciated for their healthy vitamin and mineral content and are very easy on the digestive tract. In fact, a puree of raw carrots is often recommended by naturally-oriented pediatricians to correct gastric disturbances in very young children and to improve digestion in general. Carrots are mildly diuretic, strengthen the immune system, reinforce eyesight and aid in correcting all gastrointestinal disorders in adults and children alike.

Carrots act to improve resistance to infections of all types, especially of the eyes, throat and tonsils, as well as the sinuses and the entire respiratory system.

The nutrients present in carrots stimulate the vital endocrine glands, protect the nervous system and are unequalled for increasing vim, vigor and vitality. The glands, particularly the adrenals and the hormone-secreting glands of the reproductive system, require the food elements found in carrots. Because certain forms of sterility have been traced to the over-use of over-processed foods in which vital nutrients and enzymes were destroyed, carrots have been known to overcome sterility.

Intestinal and liver complaints are often caused by a deficiency of certain elements known to be supplied by carrots. These elements act to dissolve and free unhealthy toxins clogging the system, releasing them for excretion.

New research indicates that carrots may have preventive and even curative powers in the case of cancer, particularly of the lungs. Raw carrot juice is considered a natural solvent for ulcerous and cancerous conditions. Many naturopathic doctors suggest that smokers and those with a family history of cancer may benefit by adding a cup of raw carrots or freshly squeezed carrot juice to their daily diet. Some authorities believe the preventive powers of this dietary supplement may also apply to ulcers.

For gastrointestinal catarrh, naturalists recommend you finely grate one pound of carrots, saute lightly, and dilute with half a cup of good broth. Take nothing else for the entire day. This cleansing treatment is a great help in normalizing digestion and aids the kidneys.

Carrots are particularly good as a supportive treatment for diabetics and including carrots regularly in the diet may help ease the pain of gout, rheumatism and arthritis. Premature hair loss, if caused by a vitamin deficiency, may yield to strong, regular use of grated or juiced carrots as well.

Note: Like the young mother who conquered night blindness with vast quantities of carrot juice, an intensive treatment with carrots may tend to impart a yellowish-orange tint to the skin. If this happens to you, rejoice! The condition is temporary and shows that so many toxins are being leached out of the body that the overflow is being released through the pores of the skin.

TRADITIONAL USE - EXTERNALLY: According to folk healers, just about any itching and burning skin condition may be eased with a carrot poultice. A grated raw carrot is said to accelerate the healing of ulcerated and supperating wounds of all kinds.

HOW TO PREPARE CARROTS: Carrots may be lightly cooked, but the medicinal vitamin and mineral elements are much greater in the fresh state. Well-masticated (chewed) raw carrots and grated raw carrots are equally effective, so take your choice. But please grate only what you plan on eating immediately. Grated carrots must be eaten the same day.

HOW TO PREPARE CARROT JUICE: Scrub, but don't peel, a quantity of raw carrots and run them through your juicer. The properties of carrot juice are strongest when taken immediately, so please don't hold the juice refrigerated, but enjoy it when prepared.

HOW TO PREPARE A NUTRITIOUS CARROT CEREAL: For each serving, soak 1/2 cup of Oat Flakes in cold milk overnight. The following morning, add a finely grated carrot. Warm slightly, sweeten with honey and be fortified with carrot-power for the day.

HOW TO PREPARE CARROT JAM: Scrub, but don't peal, a quantity of carrots under cold-running water. Grate finely, add enough water to barely cover, and simmer over low heat until you have a fine pulp. For each 2 cups of pulp, add the juice and grated rind of two lemons, 1/2 stick of butter and 9 ounces of sugar. Simmer the mixture until the consistency of jam, about 40 minutes. Bottle in clear glass and store refrigerated.

HOW TO PREPARE A CARROT POULTICE: Scrub a carrot well under cold-running water and grate finely onto a clean white cloth. Apply cool to the affected parts.

Chapter 7
CHAMOMILE
(Matricaria chamomilla)

Abdominal Complaints	*Diuretic*	*Mucous Membranes*
Ague	*Dropsy/Edema*	*Nervous System*
Antiseptic	*Eyes (inflamed)*	*Pain Reliever*
Anti-Inflammatory	*Fever*	*Sinus Infections*
Bowel Stimulant	*Flatulence*	*Skin Eruptions*
Change-of-Life	*Gastritis*	*Stomach Aches*
Common Cold	*Hair Conditioner*	*Testicles (inflamed)*
Complexion	*Hearing Loss*	*Tonic (general)*
Conjunctivitis	*Hemorrhoids*	*Toothache*
Cramps (menstrual)	*Laxative (mild)*	*Tranquilizer (mild)*
Diarrhea	*Limbs (paralyzed)*	*Urine (suppressed)*
Digestive Disturbances	*Menstrual Disorders*	*Wounds (open)*

PAST HISTORY: Chamomile is one of the oldest and most important of the medicinal herbs. In fact, Chamomile was so highly regarded by ancient Egyptian physicians, it was dedicated to their highest diety, the Sun God. In the Middle Ages, sweet-smelling and fragrant Chamomile was always included in the fresh straw and herbs strewn on dank castle floors to sweeten the air and cushion the feet from the rough stones, as well as being one of the premiere herbs in the medicine bag.

Chamomile's scent is similar to apples. Indeed, the name "Chamomile" comes from the Greek "ground-apple," *kamai* (on the ground) and *melon* (the Greek word for apple). In the mid-1600s, master herbalist Parkinson wrote: "Chamomile is put to divers and sundry users, both the sick and the sound, in bathing to comfort and strengthen the sound and infusions to ease pains in the sick and diseased."

DESCRIPTION & GROWING REQUIREMENTS: The single-Chamomile (Anthemis nobilis) is a low growing perennial and flourishes wild in fields, but the double-Chamomile (Matricaria chamomilla) an annual, is preferred by herbalists for its valuable properties. The

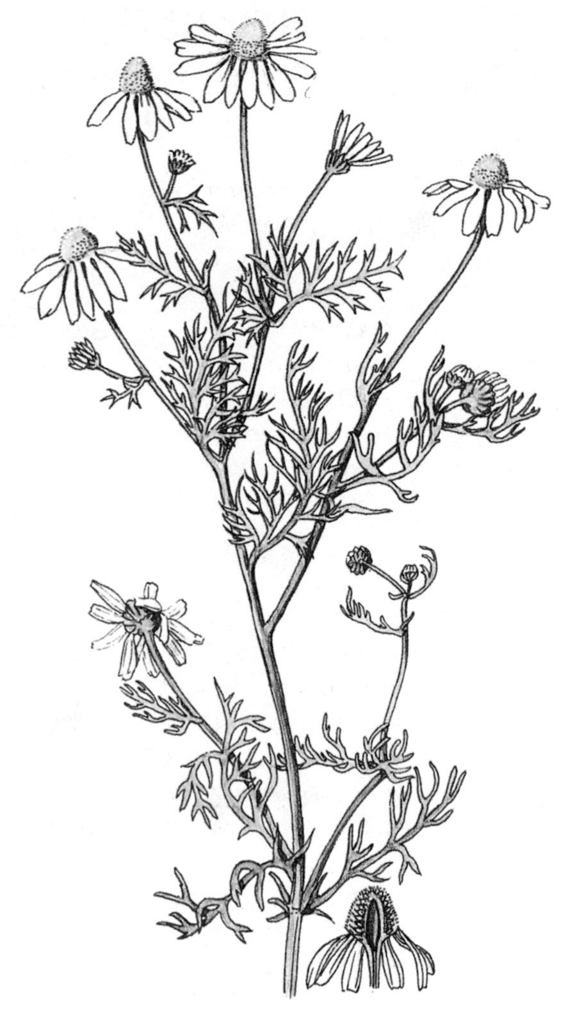

Chamomile

Matricaria chamomilla

double-Chamomile may be garden-grown from thinly sown seeds and prefers a rich loamy soil and a sunny location. Keep seedlings weed-free during early growth and you can just about forget them until harvest time.

HOW TO HARVEST & STORE: Flower-heads may be gathered from May until August when the sun is at its zenith. You may nip the flowers from the stalks with your fingernails and drop them into a clean basket, or gather them, stems and all, and scissor off the flower-heads later. To dry, place the flowers in a single layer, preferably on a screen, and put them in a dry airy place. Chamomile flowers may be used either fresh or dried.

LEGENDARY CURES: Many legends surround Chamomile, the "cure-all," especially in Europe where the use of herbs is still wide-spread. One recent tale tells of a village woman known far and wide as the "Herb Lady." A man from a neighboring village was brought to her suffering from such a severe case of dropsy (edema: an excess and abnormal accumulation of fluids in the body) that he could only sleep sitting up for fear of suffocating.

The Herb Lady knew immediately he was unable to pass urine, a fact which he confirmed. She dosed him with a glassful of Chamomile wine mornings and evenings and soon he passed an unbelievable quantity of urine. The first passing was very dark and thick, but eventually it became clear and more normal. After 8 days, the grateful villager was completely cured.

Other legends of the Herb Lady's power relate that she restored hearing loss in five persons by frying green onions in Chamomile oil, cooling it to body temperature, and dropping the strained oil into the ears frequently. She prescribed a compress made of Chamomile boiled in milk as a specific for eye pain and used Chamomile oil friction-rubs to successfully restore movement to paralyzed limbs.

TRADITIONAL USE — INTERNALLY: Chamomile is used by traditional herbalists as a tonic, diuretic, stomach aid, pain reliever, to encourage menstrual flow and as an antispasmodic. Chamomile tea is of help in cases of cramps, stomach aches, flatulence, diarrhea, all stomach and digestive disturbances and even gastritis. It assists in menstrual disorders, relieves monthly cramps, eases change-of-life problems, inflammation of the testicles, fever and all abdominal troubles.

Chamomile stimulates the peristalsis action of the bowel and is a mild laxative which works without harsh purging action. Chamomile produces copious perspiration and continues to be a useful treatment for any ague (alternate chills, fever and sweats marked by involuntary shivering or shaking, such as in malaria attacks). It is antiseptic and anti-inflammatory, both internally and externally.

Chamomile is "nature's tranquilizer." A cup of Chamomile tea calms and relaxes and acts as a mild sedative in cases of stress and nervous tension. Note: Although mild in action, Chamomile is an emmenagogue (induces menstrual flow) and should not be taken during pregnancy.

TRADITIONAL USE — EXTERNALLY: A weak Chamomile wash benefits inflamed eyes, cures conjunctivitis, relieves itching and skin eruptions and, used as a compress, can help heal open wounds. It is especially soothing in cases of inflammation of the mucous membranes and relieves a toothache when used as a mouth wash. Chamomile ointment applied directly to hemorrhoids gives wonderful relief. Chamomile steam may be inhaled to relieve colds and sinus infections. Chamomile baths benefit the entire nervous system.

As a beauty aid, a Chamomile wash of the face once weekly will soon reward you with a glowing complexion. Medieval beauties used Chamomile for shining manageable hair and some hair conditioners on the market today use Chamomile as a prime ingredient.

PREPARING CHAMOMILE TEA: Add 1 ounce of Chamomile flowers to 1 pint of boiling water and remove from heat. Allow to steep for at least 10 minutes before straining off. Note: Cover closely to prevent escape of the steam. Some of the medicinal properties of the infusion may be lost in evaporation.

PREPARING CHAMOMILE OIL: Fill a small glass bottle (not plastic) with Chamomile flowers freshly picked (or dried) and add cold-pressed olive oil slowly until the bottle is full. Close the bottle tightly and allow the oil to stand in a warm place (about 70-75 degrees F.) for two weeks. After the oil has been permeated, keep refrigerated. Before using the oil, immerse the chilled bottle in a hot-water bath until the oil is body temperature. Be careful not to allow water to seep under the lid.

PREPARING CHAMOMILE OINTMENT: Gently heat 1 cup of pure lard (not vegetable shortening) almost to boiling and add 1/2 cup fresh (or 1/4 cup dried) Chamomile flowers. As the mixture foams, stir well, but do not skim. Remove from heat, cover and let stand overnight in a cool place. The next day, heat gently until liquified and strain through cheesecloth, using the hands to squeeze out the flower heads. Stir the mass and fill a clean jelly glass or jar. Refrigerate. Employ a hot-water bath to warm before use.
Note: A tablespoon or two of cold-pressed olive oil may be added to help keep the ointment from completely solidifying under refrigeration.

PREPARING AN INHALATION: Pour a quart of boiling water over a handful of Chamomile flowers. Form a tent with large towel and breathe in the healing vapors deeply for at least 10 minutes.
Note: This treatment not only opens the sinus passages and relieves the miseries of a cold, but also benefits the skin.

PREPARING A COMPRESS: Pour 2 cups of boiling milk over a tablespoon or two of Chamomile flowers. The cloth will become very hot. Using tongs, hold the cloth above the bowl and allow to drip and cool slightly before squeezing out and applying to your patient.
Note: An old soft white cotton tee shirt, very clean, makes an excellent compress.

PREPARING A WASH: Steep two handfuls of fresh or dried Chamomile flowers in 4 quarts of boiling water for 10 minutes. Strain, and add the infusion to a full bath. For the complexion, or as a hair-conditioner, use a scant handful of Chamomile flowers steeped in a quart of boiling water and strain before use.

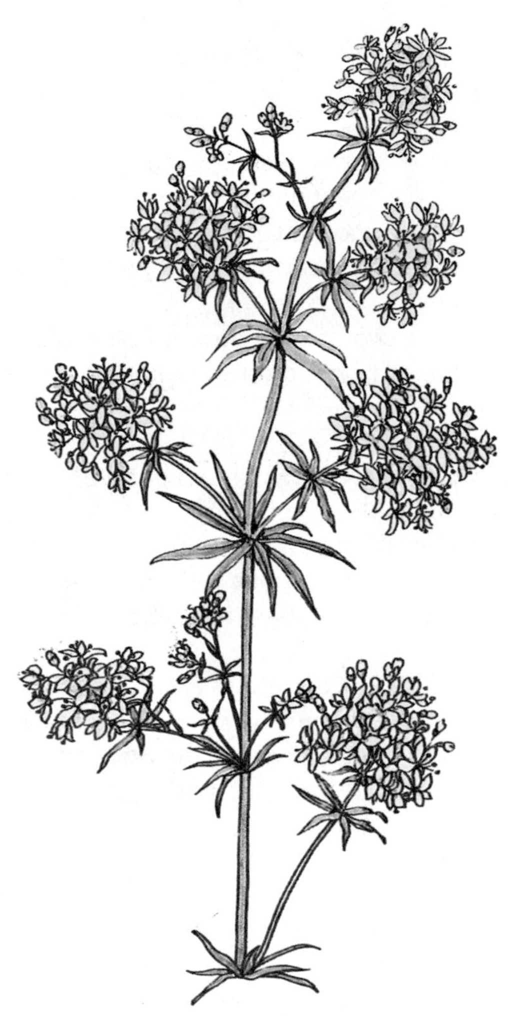

Cleavers

Galium verum

Chapter 8

CLEAVERS (Galium verum)

Anemia
Boils
Cancer (external)
Cancer (tongue)
Edema
Epilepsy
Goiter
Hysteria
Kidney Disorders
Kidney Stones
Liver Complaints
Lymphatic System
Larynx (tumor)
Muscle Spasms
Nervous Complaints
Pancreas
Skin Disorders
Spleen
Thyroid Gland
Urine (suppressed)
Wounds

PAST HISTORY: Your great-grandmother may have called the Cleaver's vine by its more old-fashioned names of Lady's Bedstraw, Maid's Hair or even Cheese Rennet, and she may have spelled it Clivers. This versatile herb was commonly used as a hair dye during the time of King Henry VII, with the leaves yielding a yellow color and the roots a reddish shade.

A very pretty legend suggests that this plant was used to make a bed for the Christ Child in the manger in Bethlehem. In later times, "bedstraw" was used as a mattress stuffing in Elizabethan England, explaining two of the common names often applied to it still.

Herbalists of the day suggested "bedstraw" for nosebleeds, internal bleeding, and used it to annoint the feet of weary travelers. It was once a prized ingredient in sheep and goat-cheese and was said to make the cheese sweeter and more pleasant to taste, hence the term "cheese rennet." American Indians used Cleavers as a healing agent for burns and wounds and master herbalists of colonial times believed it to be a remedy for kidney stones and urinary diseases.

DESCRIPTION & GROWING REQUIREMENTS: This pretty herb rewards you with clusters of small yellow flowers from June to September and has leaves in rings of six around its stem. Cleavers can be best established by dividing the roots in the spring after the plant is growing well.

This plant spreads readily and will crowd out weeds in its bed, making cultivation easy. Be warned, however. Cleavers doesn't always stay where you want it and will encroach on other plantings nearby. It isn't very fussy as to its environment and will do nicely in full sun or even partial shade and can tolerate a poor soil, as long as it is in a well-drained location.

HOW TO HARVEST & STORE: The entire plant may be used and the best time for harvesting Cleavers is in July when the medicinal qualities are most potent. After the flowers have bloomed, gather whole stalks, bundle them together and hang the bundles upside down to dry in an airy place.

Roots may be gathered when the plant is dormant, preferably in early spring or late autumn. Brush off as much earth as possible, but don't wash. Put the roots in a warm airy place to dry for future use.

LEGENDARY CURES: Since the introduction of iodized salt into the modern diet, goiters (an abnormal growth of the thyroid gland) have apparently disappeared in America. However, I still remember my grandmother in Bavaria treating a friend with warm tea made with the fresh-pressed juice of the Cleavers plant. Following grandmother's instructions, the woman gargled as deeply as possible and was overjoyed to find that her disfiguring goiter gradually grew smaller until it was completely gone.

A very sad story with a happy ending tells of a man, Otto K., afflicted with a serious kidney disorder in which one kidney finally was surgically removed. Mr. K.'s one remaining kidney was not functioning normally and the doctors were unable to correct his condition. After drinking four cups of Cleavers tea with Goldenrod (see Chapter 14) and Yellow Dead Nettle (see Chapter 34) daily for some time, the fortunate gentleman found his kidney complaint completely cured.

At least one botanical authority, Richard Willfort, suggests that rinsing the mouth and sipping Cleavers tea may well clear up cancer of the tongue. Willfort also believes the freshly pressed juice of Cleavers can be mixed with butter to make an ointment which may help external cancerous growths and which may possibly clear cancer-like skin disorders.

Although scientists do not agree and can find no reason why it should be so, a reliable source reports that Cleavers helped a woman in her 60s, Ruth C., who had developed a tumor in her larynx. Mrs. C. was operated on unsuccessfully and by the time six months had passed, her pain became unbearable. She was without feeling or movement in her left arm and hand. A second operation was scheduled in which the surgeon planned to sever the nerves to free her from the worst of the pain.

On the recommendation of an herbal authority, Mrs. C. began drinking Cleavers tea with Calendula (see Chapter 5), Yarrow (see Chapter 33), and Stinging Nettle (see Chapter 28) and gargling with it as well. The terrible pain vanished after just four days on this mixture and she regained feeling in her arm and hand. To the amazement of the doctor, the second operation was unnecessary. The astounded physician recommended the woman continue with the herbal treatment. I understand Mrs. C. is now completely well and is very happy to be able to handle her daily chores again.

TRADITIONAL USE — INTERNALLY: Cleavers tea is traditionally recommended for ridding the liver, kidneys, pancreas and spleen of toxic wastes. This powerful cleansing herb is said to stimulate the lymphatic system and is helpful in cases of anemia and edema and can even relieve the most stubborn 'charley-horse' or muscle-spasm.

Many herbalists believe Cleavers is of benefit to the epileptic, in cases of hysteria, nervous complaints, suppressed urine and kidney stones. There are many reports in herbal lore of Cleavers normalizing an imbalance of the thyroid gland as well.

TRADITIONAL USE — EXTERNALLY: Cleavers is wonderfully beneficial to the skin. When the tea is used as a wash, it clears many skin disorders and speeds healing of wounds and boils. When the freshly pressed juice of Cleavers is dabbed on the skin, it assists in removing blackheads and tightens and tones at the same time.

PREPARING CLEAVERS TEA: Pour 1 pint of boiling water over 1 heaping teaspoon of Cleavers. Cover and allow to steep for 5 minutes.

PREPARING FRESH JUICE: Gather a generous quantity of fresh Cleavers (leaves, stems & flowers) and wash carefully. While still wet, place in a juice extractor.

PREPARING AN OINTMENT: When you have extracted 1/4 cup of fresh juice, stir into it about 1/8th pound of sweet butter (room temperature) to make a paste. Store in refrigerator.

Chapter 9
CLUB MOSS
(Lycopodium clavatum)

Bedsores	*Gout*	*Renal Colic*
Blood Pressure	*Joints (deformed)*	*Reproductive Organs*
Breath (shortness of)	*Kidneys*	*Rheumatism*
Chafing	*Kidneys (stones)*	*Skin Diseases*
Constipation	*Liver*	*Sores (open)*
Eczema/Erysipelas	*Liver (cirrhosis)*	*Testes (inflamed)*
Extremities (cramped)	*Muscle Spasms*	*Urinary Tract*
Diarrhea	*Piles/Hemorrhoids*	*Urine (suppressed)*

PAST HISTORY: Ancient physicians dried and used the entire plant as a stomachic and diuretic for stones and other kidney complaints. In the 17th century, the spores of this herb were used as a diuretic in dropsy and cases of urine suppression, against chronic diarrhea and dysentery and as a nervine in muscle spasms. Club Moss was once used against the hydrophobia caused by the bite of a mad dog, somewhat successfully if old accounts can be credited.

Club Moss was much used in Europe in days of old, although it never earned a place in the London Pharmacopeia. However, a tincture of Club Moss appeared in the U.S. Pharmacopeia once upon a time prescribed for 'irritability of the bladder.'

DESCRIPTION & GROWING REQUIREMENTS: As its name suggests, this is a mossy trailing plant which puts forth ramblers that cling to the ground with tiny hair-like roots. The ramblers eventually develop high forked branches which are yielding to the touch. Only after the plants are 4 years old do they develop the spike-like yellowish pods which provide the pollen we term "Club Moss powder."

This species of Club Moss grows all over the world, but the spores are harvested commercially, mainly in Russia, Germany and Switzerland. If the plant is exposed to direct sunlight, it withers and shrivels, preferring instead the shade of the forest. Since I have been unable to find a source for this plant, I believe the only way to propagate it in the home garden is to beg a cutting from someone who is lucky enough to

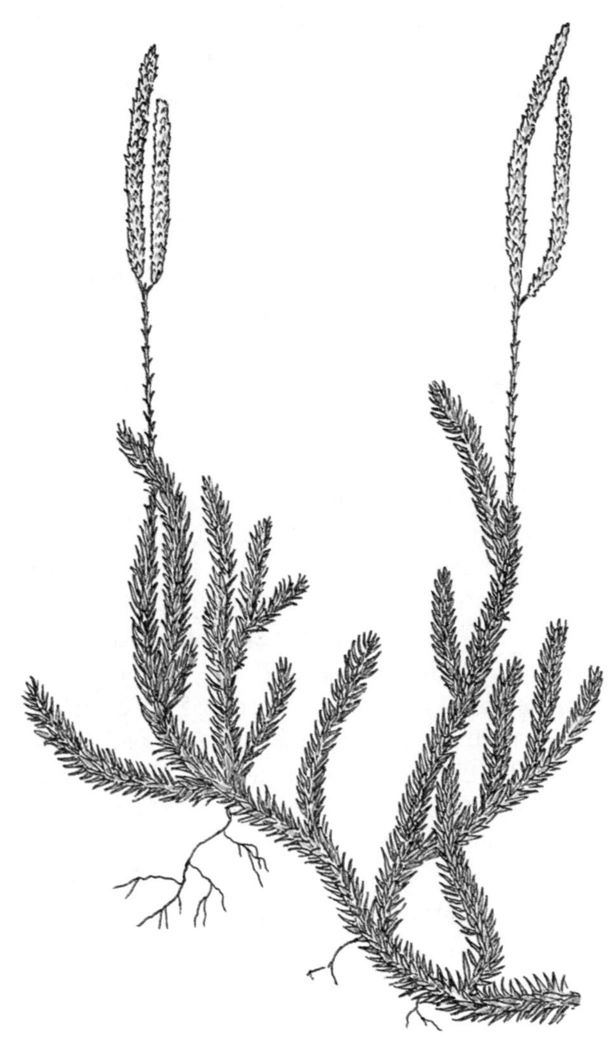

Club Moss

Lycopodium clavatum

have it established.

HOW TO HARVEST & STORE: As the spikes of the Club Moss reach maturity, usually during July and August, the tops are cut and the powder is shaken out from the pods and sifted.

LEGENDARY CURES: Even after the modern physician has given up in cases of severe cirrhosis of the liver, Club Moss may sometimes work the most amazing cures. One serious effect of the last stages of this ailment is a debilitating shortness of breath, particularly during the night. Robert A., suffering from terminal involvement of the liver and drawing every breath with effort, was treated with Club Moss. After taking just 1 cup of Club Moss tea, Mr. A. reports his breathing was eased and the awful nightly shortness of breath he experienced disappeared. Not surprisingly, the active principle of Club Moss is radium. You will be doing anyone suffering shortness of breath a real service by telling them about Club Moss.

In cases of urine suppression, Club Moss tea promotes the most copious flow and is an unparallelled natural diuretic. Applied externally, a small cheesecloth bag of Club Moss is placed in the area of the bladder. Louise J. had to be hospitalized again and again because she was unable to urinate normally due to severe cramps of this vital organ. The Club Moss bag did the trick and Mrs. J. always tries this method before submitting to hospitalization.

My own wife finds that she can control her high blood pressure, caused by overfunctioning of her kidneys, by applying a bag of Club Moss to the kidney region overnight every so often. I know this is effective. Her blood pressure dropped from 210 to 160 and her doctor is amazed she no longer needs her medication.

Many people all over the world have been relieved of cramping of the extremities and even cramps caused by huge scars of healed wounds or surgical operations which can twist the underlying muscles cruelly. For instance, Allen E., a disabled soldier, suffered awfully from an immense scar which almost covered his back. His pain was so severe that he broke out in perspiration all over. Mr. E. tried Club Moss baths and the application of a Club Moss pillow. Much to his relief, the pain he had been experiencing for so many years disappeared.

Another interesting story concerning the power of Club Moss occurred some years ago when I was on a climbing expedition in

Austria, but I've never forgotten it. One of the climbers was enjoying the rarified air of the mountains and jokingly wound his hat with a Club Moss rambler. When we returned to camp, another member of the expedition suddenly doubled over and fell to the ground with the most terrible muscle spasm in his leg. Nothing helped. Someone suggested winding the Club Moss rambler around the leg and we all laughed, but the pain was so excruciating that my friend decided to try it. In just a few minutes, his muscles straightened out and let go and he was able to walk normally without pain.

We were all very impressed and I brought home some ramblers for my grandmother, who continually complained of cramping in her legs. She was delighted to find they gave her almost immediate relief.

TRADITIONAL USE — INTERNALLY: Club Moss tea is recommended for easing and healing the pain of gout, rheumatism, piles and deformed joints of all kinds. Chronic constipation can be cured by drinking the tea and diarrhea can be halted. However, in cases of diarrhea, only a little should be taken as it may possibly cause cramping of the intestines.

Club Moss tea is beneficial for involvement of the urinary tract and reproductive organs, for inflammations of the testes and kidney stones and helps with renal colic. Inflammation of the liver, cirrhosis of the liver and tumors, even if malignant, often yield to Club Moss tea.

TRADITIONAL USE — EXTERNALLY: By far, the most widespread use of Club Moss is as a dusting powder in various skin diseases, such as eczema and erysipelas and for excoriated surfaces of the skin of all kinds. Bedsores of bed-ridden invalids yield to Club Moss powder and open sores of all kinds are relieved quickly by the gentle application of Club Moss powder. Club Moss powder is a time-honored specific against chafing in infants as well. An interesting characteristic of this powder is that once the hands are well-covered, the skin remains dry even if they are dipped in water.

PREPARING CLUB MOSS TEA: Pour 1 pint of boiling water over a level teaspoon of Club Moss. Steep for 5 minutes and strain. Sip 1 cupful on an empty stomach half an hour before breakfast. In cases of cirrhosis or malignancy of the liver, try 2 cupfuls daily.

PREPARING A CLUB MOSS PILLOW: One, two or even three handfuls of dried Club Moss, depending on the size of the cramped area, may be stuffed into a pillow of any lightweight material. Apply overnight for amazing relief. A pillow thus prepared retains its potency for a year.

PREPARING A CLUB MOSS SITZ BATH: Steep a generous quantity of dried Club Moss overnight in cold water. Strain the next morning, warm slightly and add the mixture to your sitz bath.

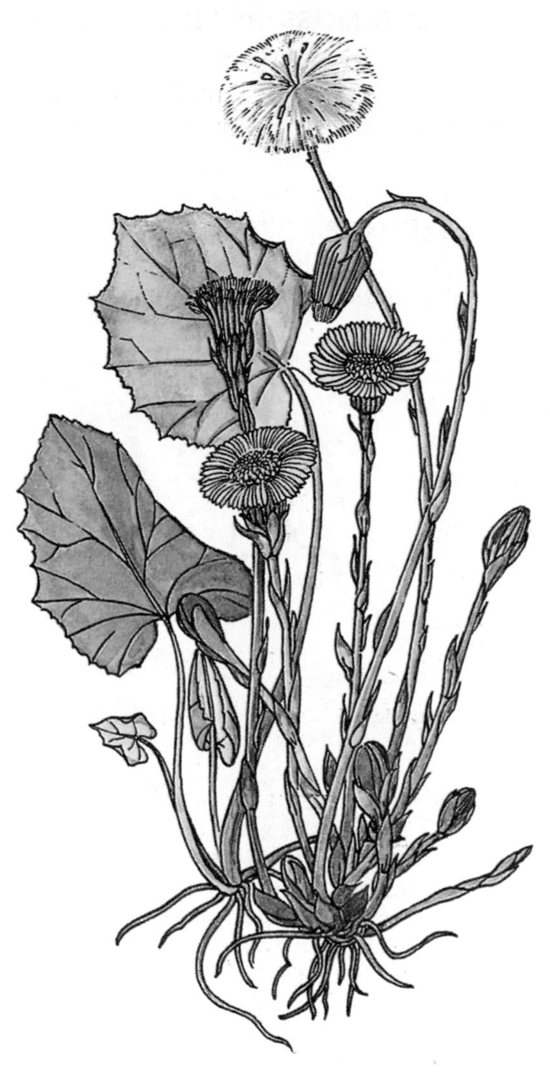

Coltsfoot

Tussilago farfara

Chapter 10
COLTSFOOT
(Tussilago farfara)

Asthma
Breath (shortness of)
Bronchitis
Bruises
Bursitis
Cough
Earache
Erysipelas
Hoarseness
Laryngitis
Pharyngitis
Phlebitis
Pleurisy
Pneumonia
Smokers Aid
Sores (scrofulous)
Tuberculosis (early)

PAST HISTORY: Coltsfoot has always been an important part of the herbal physician's pharmacopeia. In Paris, Coltsfoot was the symbol of the apothecary, with its distinctive flowers being painted on the doorpost of the shop to signify the pharmacist within.

Master Herbalist Culpepper wrote: "The fresh leaves or juice or syrup of Coltsfoot is good for a bad, dry cough or wheezing and shortness of breath. The dry leaves are best for those who have their rheums and distillations upon their lungs causing a cough, for which also the dried leaves taken as tobacco, or the root is very good."

Coltsfoot is considered nature's best help for the lungs. Smoking the leaves for a persistent cough is recommended by many herbal authorities, both ancient and modern. In fact, Coltsfoot leaves form the base of British Herb Tobacco said to relieve the asthmatic and the labored breathing of those afflicted with chronic bronchitis.

DESCRIPTION & GROWING REQUIREMENTS: One of the peculiarities of Coltsfoot is that the flowers and leaves appear at different times during the season. Even before the first signs of spring while there is still a chill in the air, Coltsfoot sends forth its stalk of golden flowers, as early as February in some climates. In fact, it is the Coltsfoot flower that offers the bees and other honey-sipping insects their first nectar of the year. Oddly enough, its leaves, green on the upper surface and fuzzed with silver underneath, do not appear until the flower heads begin to wither, usually sometime in May. Coltsfoot obliges us by growing happily in stiff clay and flourishes wild in wet ground and wastelands. It may be grown from seed.

HOW TO HARVEST & STORE: Coltsfoot leaves offer stronger medicinal properties than do the flowers. Plan to gather first the flower heads and then the leaves as they make their respective appearances. Snip off the flowers by hand and drop into a basket. Do the same with the leaves and spread both in a single layer, preferably on a screen so air can circulate, and place in a dry airy place.

Dig out the roots only when the plant is dormant, during very early spring or late fall. Brush off the earth clinging to them without washing and put them aside to dry also.

LEGENDARY CURES: To cure an obstinate cough, the renowned Pliny himself recommended the dried leaves and roots of Coltsfoot be burned and the smoke inhaled deeply into the mouth through a reed and then swallowed. The sufferer was directed to sip a little wine between swallows of smoke. Pliny cautioned that the full benefit of the Coltsfoot smoke was only achieved if the burning was done on a bed of cypress charcoal.

The botanical name of Coltsfoot, "Tussilago," itself means "cough dispeller." The British Pharmacopeia directs that both the flower-stalks and the leaves be employed in the preparation of Syrup of Coltsfoot, much recommended for treatment of chronic bronchitis.

TRADITIONAL USE - INTERNALLY: Herbalists, both ancient and modern, agree that Coltsfoot, with pectoral and anti-inflammatory properties, can be used successfully as treatment for bronchitis, laryngitis, pharyngitis, asthma and pleurisy. In cases of early tuberculosis, Coltsfoot has been known to be of benefit. Coltsfoot tea, hot and liberally sweetened with honey, can clear a persistent cough and conquer hoarseness when taken frequently during the day.

The smoker, the asthmatic and those suffering with bronchitis will find relief by using 2 or 3 teaspoons of fresh-pressed juice of the Coltsfoot leaves, rich in Vitamin C, stirred into a cup of warm broth or milk. An inhalation of Coltsfoot steam assists in chronic bronchitis and all cases of shortness of breath.

TRADITIONAL USE - EXTERNALLY: A Coltsfoot poultice may be applied directly in cases of pneumonia, erysipelas and to bruises where swelling and discoloration are present. This eases the pain of bursitis as well. The effect of a Coltsfoot poultice is amazingly strong.

The inflammation and pain of phlebitis is relieved by a Coltsfoot poultice applied and lightly bandaged to hold it in place. A compress aids healing of stubborn scrofulous sores. The fresh-pressed juice of the leaves, lightly warmed in a water-bath, can be dropped into the ear to ease an earache.

PREPARING COLTSFOOT TEA: Pour 1 pint of boiling water over a mixture of flowers and leaves and steep, closely covered, for 5 minutes. Strain before use.

PREPARING A COUGH EXPECTORANT: Mix equal parts of the leaves and flowers of Coltsfoot, Lungwort and Plantain (see Chapter 23). Pour 1 pint of boiling water over 2 tablespoons of the blended herbs and steep, covered, for 10 minutes. Sweeten with honey to taste and sip 3 cups of this tea daily as hot as is comfortable.

PREPARING FRESH-PRESSED JUICE: Gather a goodly quantity of fresh Coltsfoot leaves and wash gently in running water. While still wet, put the leaves through a juice extractor.

PREPARING A POULTICE: Gather a quantity of fresh Coltsfoot leaves, wash gently and crush onto a clean cloth with the back of a spoon. Apply directly to the affected area.

PREPARING A COMPRESS: Pour 1 quart of boiling water over a double handful of the flowers and leaves. Steep, covered, for 15 minutes. Cool slightly before wringing out a clean white cloth and applying to the painful area.

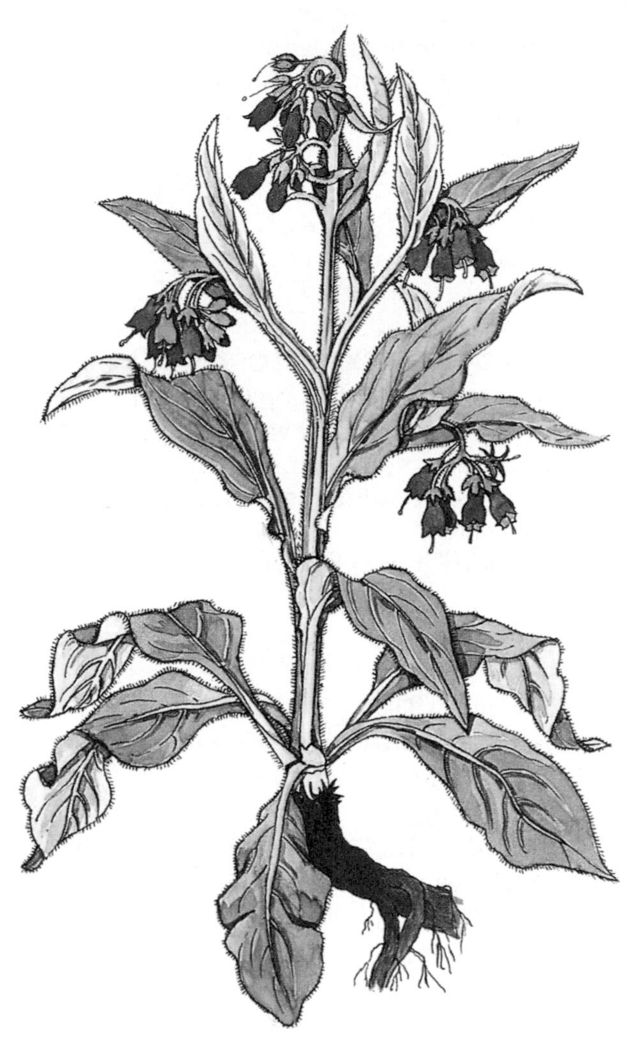

Comfrey

Symphytum officinale

Chapter 11
COMFREY
(Symphytum officinale)

Arthritis	*Gout*	*Pleghm (tough)*
Bronchitis	*Injuries*	*Pleurisy*
Bone Bruises	*Intestines (bleeding)**	*Rheumatism*
Bone Fractures	*Joint (infected)*	*Shock*
Bruises	*Joint (swollen)*	*Sprains*
Bursitis	*Limbs (amputated)*	*Stomach Problems**
Digestive Disorders	*Limbs (paralyzed*	*Varicose Veins*
Disc (slipped)	*Neck (stiff)*	*Varicose Ulcers*
Dislocation	*Over-Exertion*	*Wounds*

**Comfrey may be taken against intestinal bleeding (and stomach problems), as long as cancer is not present. See your doctor if bleeding does not stop quickly. Do not take Comfrey over a prolonged period of time.*

PAST HISTORY: No herb garden or apothecary shop of the past was complete without Comfrey. In the Middle Ages, Comfrey was renowned and called "Knit Bone" and Boneset" by country folk. Its common name is a corruption of *con firma,* an allusion to its effect in firming broken bones. The botanical name "Symphytum" comes from the Greek *symphyo* and means "to unite."

In his writings, Master Herbalist Culpepper says, "The great Comfrey restrains spitting of blood. The root boiled in water or wine and the decoction drank, heals inward hurts, bruises, wounds and ulcers of the lungs and causes the phlegm that oppresses to be easily spit forth."

A Madam Susanna Avery in "May ye 12th Anno Domini 1688," has this to say: "Comfrey - A Wound Herb - The roots heal all inwarde woundes and burstings."

The British Medical Journal of 1912 reported that the active properties of Comfrey were from the Allantoin it contains and stated "Allantoin in aqueous solution has a powerful action in strengthening epithelial formation and is a valuable remedy for external ulcerations and ulcers of the stomach and duodenum."

It appears that, in the case of Comfrey at least, the scientific community and the herbalists were in agreement.

DESCRIPTION & GROWING REQUIREMENTS: Comfrey grows in clumps and can reach a height of three feet. It thrives in either full sun or partial shade and is propagated from root cuttings or transplants. Comfrey has large fuzzy dark green leaves, rough and pointed at the ends, and develops pale pink bell-like flowers. It likes a lot of moisture and makes a very pretty addition to the herb garden. Comfrey is a perennial and dies back in cold weather to reappear in the spring.

HOW TO HARVEST & STORE: Pinch the young leaves from the herb as they appear for fresh use. You may dry some for future use. Lay them on a screen so air can circulate around them and put the screen in a warm, dry place. The roots, about the thickness of your thumb, should be harvested when the plant is dormant, either in very early spring or late fall.

The plant benefits and may be kept tidy by root division, so don't fear harming it by harvesting the root. Brush off the clinging earth, but don't wash, and store in a dry place. A root several years old may be almost black on the outside, but will be sticky and moist within. If you wish, you may chop or grind the fresh root and then dry.

LEGENDARY CURES: Several years ago, a young woman by the name of Melanie N. was in an automobile accident and suffered a fracture of her right hip. The surgeon found it necessary to insert a pin and she went home with no pain and no difficulty whatsoever in walking or moving around. Because Melanie was young and healthy, she forgot all about the pin and neglected going in for the necessary check-up. Unfortunately, this neglect led to a bone infection that eventually caused great pain and she hurried in to the doctor. He removed the pin and gave her injections of a strong antibiotic for the infection and pain pills to dull her agony, but the bone failed to heal and the pain continued. Melanie was in quite an awful state when a neighbor prepared a warm poultice of Comfrey root from her own small stock and applied it to the infected joint.

Melanie said it was almost a miracle how her pain disappeared overnight! The relief she gained was indescribable and the next day she was able to move freely without pain. Fearing to stop the treatment, she secured some roots herself from an herbal shop, dried them in her oven on low heat, ground them finely and prepared her own poultices from then on.

In cases of over-exertion, dislocation, shock or sprain where limbs paralyzed, a poultice of scalded Comfrey leaves has been known to effect a cure. Whitney Y., a lumberjack, had all but lost the use of his arm because the socket was so inflammed and sore. The doctor prescribed a long rest, but the man had to work to support his family and was at a loss as to what to do. In despair, his wife rubbed a tincture of Comfrey into the joint several times a day and to Mr. Y.'s surprise, the complaint eased and the pain disappeared after just a few days.

To this day, country folk believe that the gnarled knobs which form painfully on the joints of the hands, elbows and feet of the arthritic can be eased and in some cases made to disappear by the application of Comfrey poultices.

TRADITIONAL USE - INTERNALLY: Comfrey root tea, 2 to 4 cups daily, is traditionally used in cases of bleeding in the stomach, disorders of the digestive system, against the pain of pleurisy and to bring up the pleghm formed in chronic bronchitis. In the case of stomach ulcers, a tea combining Comfrey, Calendula (see Chapter 5) and Knot Grass is beneficial.

An old European recipe calls for the young leaves of Comfrey to be dipped in a light batter and fried in oil.

TRADITIONAL USE - EXTERNALLY: Warm poultices made from the Comfrey root can ease varicose ulcers, rheumatism, swollen joints, gout, stiff neck and the pain occuring in amputated limbs. As a compress, a Comfrey tincture is effective against wounds, injuries of all kinds, bruises and even bone fractures.

A sitz bath prepared with Comfrey leaves is excellent for stimulating the sluggish circulation which causes varicose veins, the pain of a slipped disc or bone bruises and can immediately ease the suffering of rheumatism or bursitis.

PREPARING COMFREY ROOT TEA: Soak 2 heaping teaspoons of the finely chopped root in a pint of cold water overnight. Warm slightly in the morning, strain, and sip. Note: Comfrey is prepared as a cold infusion only and must not be steeped in boiling water.

PREPARING COMFREY TEA FOR STOMACH ULCERS: Combine 2 parts of Comfrey root and 1 part each of Calendula and Knot Grass. Take 1 heaping teaspoon of the blend and pour 1 cup of boiling water over the mixture. Cover and allow to steep for three minutes. Strain and sip 3 to 4 cups during the day.

PREPARING A COMFREY TINCTURE: Wash and clean the Comfrey root with a brush. Chop finely, place in a glass bottle and cover with whiskey or fruit spirits. Keep the bottle in a warm place (70-75 degrees F.) for two weeks before use.

PREPARING COMFREY WINE: Wash and clean the Comfrey root with a brush. Chop finely and steep in a pint of white wine for at least six weeks. Comfrey wine is considered an excellent remedy for pulmonary complaints.

PREPARING A COMFREY ROOT POULTICE: Wash, clean and chop the root finely. Dry well in a low oven and grind into a meal. Mix quickly with very hot water and add a few drops of cold-pressed olive oil. Spread the poultice on a clean white cloth and apply warm to the affected area. Bandage lightly to hold in place.

PREPARING FRESH COMFREY LEAVES FOR APPLICATION: Gather a quantity of fresh leaves and crush them into a pulp with the back of a heavy spoon. Apply to the affected area.

PREPARING HOT COMFREY LEAVES: Gather the fresh leaves and scald with boiling water. Apply warm to the affected area.

PREPARING COMFREY ROOT OINTMENT: Wash, clean, and finely chop about 4 to 6 fresh Comfrey roots. Add to 2 cups of heated, lard (not vegetable shortening) and cool overnight. Gently heat the mixture the next morning and press through a cheesecloth to remove the residue of the root. Pour into small clean jars and store in the refrigerator. 2 or 3 tablespoons of cold-pressed olive oil may be added to help keep the mixture soft. Note: Comfrey root ointment may be used in place of the ground root for treatment of wounds in humans or animals.

PREPARING A COMFREY LEAF BATH: Soak 2 handfuls of fresh or dried Comfrey leaves overnight in 2 quarts of cold water. Bring the mixture to a boil the following day, strain, and add to the bath water. Note: For a sitz bath, use one handful of leaves in 1 quart of water and proceed as above.

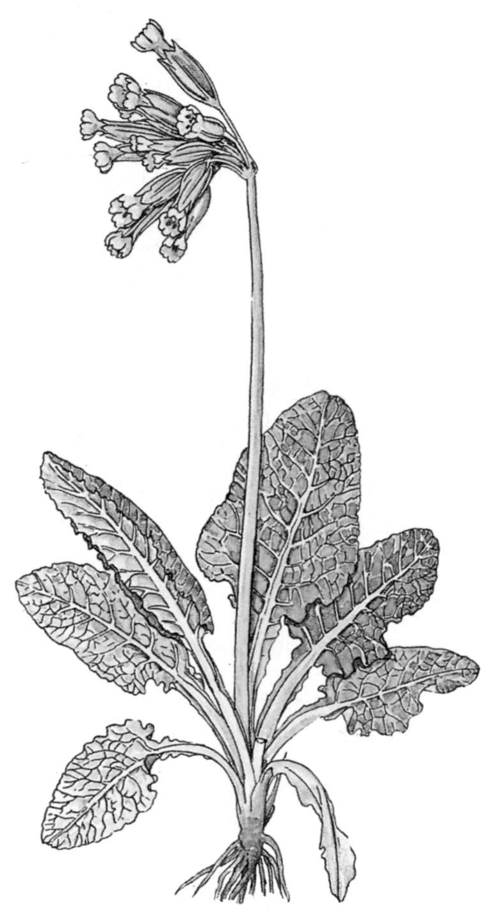

Cowslip

Primula officinalis

Chapter 12
COWSLIP
(Primula officinalis)

Bladder	*Gout*	*Kidney (stones)*
Blood (purifier)	*Heart (inflammation)*	*Nervous Disorders*
Complexion Aid	*Heart (strengther)*	*Rheumatism Stroke*
Diuretic	*Insomnia*	

PAST HISTORY: In *A Midsummer Night's Dream*, Shakespeare wrote: "In their gold coats, spots you see. These be rubies fairy favours; In those freckles lie their savours." With these words, the immortal bard was referring to the old belief that the Cowslip flower had magical powers for improving the complexion.

The ladies of Elizabethan England believed Cowslip wine or ointment 'taketh away spots and wrinkles from the face.' Master Herbalist Culpepper said, "Our city dames know well enough the ointment or distilled water of it adds beauty or at least restores it when lost." When taken internally, Culpepper's writings report, "The flowers preserved or conserved and a quantity the size of a nutmeg taken every morning is a sufficient dose for inward diseases, but for wounds, spots, wrinkles and sunburnings, an ointment is made of the leaves and hog's lard."

In the 16th century, the powdered roots of Cowslip were boiled in ale by country folk and the resultant potent drink used for dizziness, insomnia or other nervous complaints.

DESCRIPTION & GROWING REQUIREMENTS: There is nothing prettier in early spring than a meadow full of Cowslips swaying in the sunshine. The Cowslip bears golden yellow *umbels*, a cluster of flowers arising from a single stem, centered in a perfect rosette of leaves. The Cowslip is commonly seen on mountain slopes and in pastures and has a faint honey-like fragrance.

Another variety, Primula elatior, known as the Tall Cowslip, has the same medicinal value as Primula officinalis. Many nurseries carry the Cowslip as a potted plant, which you may successfully transplant into your herb garden.

HOW TO HARVEST & STORE: Although old herbalists sometimes employed the leaves and roots of the Cowslip, most authorities today use only the flowers themselves. However, Cowslip root tea does assist in expelling stones and instruction for its use is given in the text.

Harvest the flower umbels in late spring when they appear in profusion. Spread them out on a screen and place in a warm airy place to dry thoroughly. The roots may be dug in very early spring or late autumn and dried on a screen also.

LEGENDARY CURES: A renowned herbalist tells the story of Ralph D. who was forced to take strong sleeping draughts prescribed by his physician in order to get just a wink of sleep every night. This very sad state of affairs had continued for many, many years and the man was in a highly nervous state. Mr. D.'s main problem was a sharp stabbing pain that commenced in one foot and shot clear up his leg every time he tried to lie down. Indeed, his system was so dependent on drug-induced sleep that the herbalist himself doubted he could be helped by natural means.

However, Ralph D. was desperate and begged to try the special Cowslip tea the herbalist blended for insomnia. The herbalist agreed and supplied him with a quantity of the blend and instructions for its use. Within a week, Mr. D. returned with the happy news that he was not only sleeping well for the first time in years, but the strange pain in his foot, arising from his nervous condition, and which had plagued him for so long had disappeared as well!

TRADITIONAL USE - INTERNALLY: As the example given above so well demonstrates, Cowslip tea promotes healthy natural sleep and conquers nervous disorders of all kinds.

Cowslip tea is traditionally recommended for strengthening the heart and is considered an excellent aid for soothing inflammation of the heart muscle itself, dropsy, and may prevent strokes. Dried and powdered Cowslip roots can help expel kidney and bladder stones when used as a tea liberally sweetened with raw honey. Cowslip remains the prime ingredient in many spring tonics and has blood cleansing properties which assist the body in removing the toxins which lead to gout and rheumatism. Both these painful conditions yield to 1 or 2 cups of Cowslip tea taken daily for a lengthy period.

My grandmother made a quantity of Cowslip wine every spring for medicinal purposes and dried both the roots and flowers against future need. Along with the garlic she insisted be taken, we all had our Cowslip tea.

TRADITIONAL USE - EXTERNALLY: In spite of diligent research, I have been unable to find an authoritative source who recommends Cowslip ointment or wine as an aid to a clear complexion. However, if Shakespeare may be believed, you might try a cotton pad dipped in Cowslip wine patted on a clean face for a few weeks to see if the beauties of the past were right.

PREPARING COWSLIP TEA FOR INSOMNIA: Blend together 2 tablespoons Cowslip, 1 tablespoon Lavender, 2 teaspoons St. John's Wort (see Chapter 29), 3 teaspoons Hops, and 1/2 teaspoon Valerian roots. For 1 cup of tea, take one heaping teaspoonful of the blend and pour a cup of boiling water over the mixture. Steep covered for three or four minutes. Strain and sip very warm before going to bed. Sweeten with a little raw honey, if you like.

PREPARING COWSLIP SPRING-TONIC: This special blending of herbs is noted for its blood-cleansing properties. Mix together 2 tablespoons Cowslip, 2 tablespoons Elder flowers, 3 teaspoons Stinging Nettle (see Chapter 28), and 3 teaspoons Dandelion roots (see Chapter 13). Pour 1 cup of boiling water over a heaping teaspoon of the blend and steep, covered, for three or four minutes. Strain, sweeten with honey, if desired, and sip.

PREPARING COWSLIP WINE: Cowslip wine requires fresh flowers and therefore is traditionally made in the spring. Fill a quart glass bottle loosely with fresh umbels and add white wine to completely cover all the blossoms. Keep the bottle in a warm place (70-75 degrees F.) for two weeks, but do not cork tightly. Allow a little air to circulate within. For heart problems, three tablespoons daily are recommended, or take a sip now and again as needed for nervous complaints.

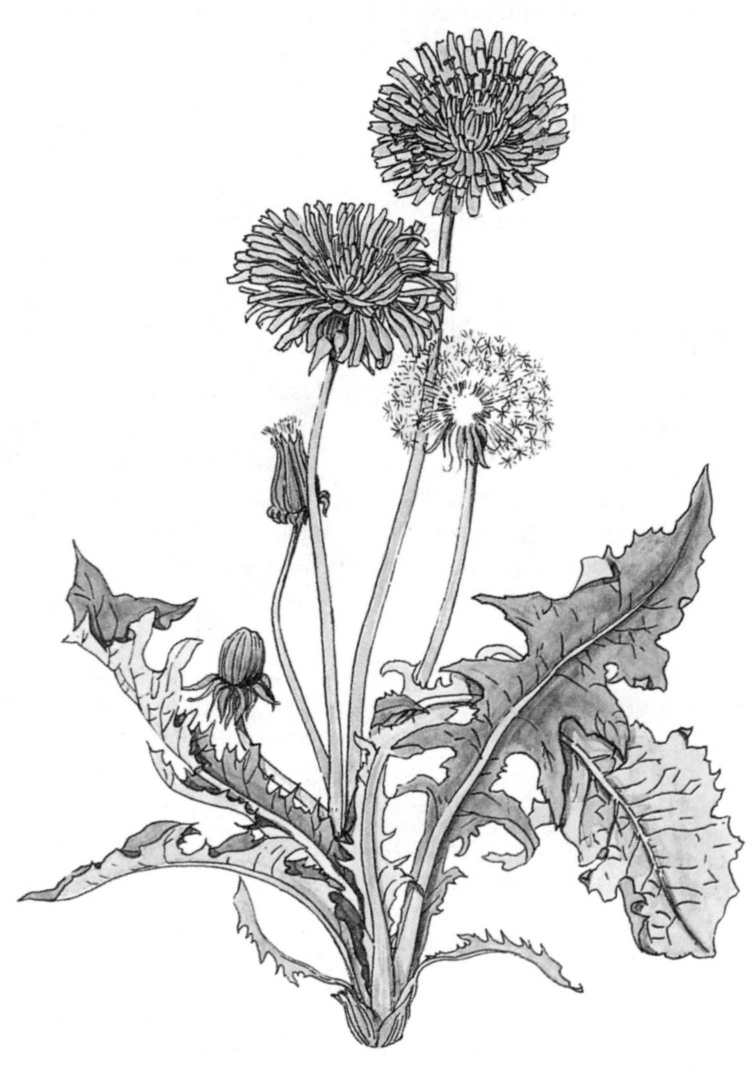

Dandelion

Taraxacum officinale

Chapter 13
DANDELION
(Taraxacum officinale)

Blood (purifier)
Blood (detoxifier)
Diabetes
Digestive Tract
Energizer
Exhaustion
Glands (swollen)
Gout
Jaundice
Liver Complaints
Liver (inflamed)
Metabolic Aid
Rheumatism
Spleen Disorders

PAST HISTORY: It is believed the deep jagged cuts of the Dandelion leaf, which resemble the teeth of the King of Beasts, gave this herb its name. In ages past, the French called it *Dent de lion* (teeth of the Lion); the original Latin name was *Dens leonis* and the Greeks called it *Leontodon.* An herbal written in 1485 concludes with the following statement: "The Herb was much employed by Master Wilhelmus, a surgeon, who on account of its virtues, likened it to 'eynem lewen zan, genannt zu latin Dens leonis.' (a lion's tooth, called in Latin Dens leonis).

The first written record of this remarkable herb appears in writings of 10th and 11th century Arabian physicians, who considered it a type of endive. Welsh papers dating back to the 13th century praise the Dandelion. The herbalists of medieval Europe valued the Dandelion for its medicinal properties and apothecaries of the day dug the roots personally, pressed the juice and sold the extract. The British Pharmacopeia directed the root be collected only between September and February because the juice was thought to be more potent during these months. Interestingly enough, the U.S. Pharmacopeia officially recognized the dried root, but not the extracted juice.

Dandelion wine, beer, and even Dandelion stout were enjoyed by the country folk and a Dandelion coffee, made from the dried, roasted and ground root, still made today, is said to taste much like regular coffee and is more wholesome.

DESCRIPTION & GROWING REQUIREMENTS: No matter where you live, if you look outside in the spring, you are apt to see the sunny yellow heads of the Dandelion beautifying the landscape, or perhaps infesting the lawn to your dismay, depending on your point of view. This potent medicinal herb is often regarded as a troublesome weed and is very difficult to discourage. The Dandelion has a thick, long tap root, dark on the outside and white within. The leaves rise directly from the root and form a rosette around the radius of the plant and a single stem bears the familiar golden blossom. The Dandelion self-seeds as the flower turns into a puff ball and its tiny seeds are blown by the wind to spring up everywhere.

HOW TO HARVEST & STORE: The very young fresh leaves and stems should be gathered in early spring before the plant flowers. They make a delightful addition to salads and, like endive, have a slightly bitter taste but are juicy and delicious nonetheless. Country folk still enjoy a healthy 'mess of Dandelion greens' cooked lightly with potatoes and perhaps a piece of bacon.

The flowers themselves should be gathered in the early summer when the fields are full of the dancing butter-yellow blossoms. I remember my grandmother and the hired girl coming in with aprons brimming over with the golden flowers. This meant a treat was in store for the whole family. Grandmother made a delicious Dandelion honey. (See recipe below.)

The roots should be dug out in early spring or late fall when the plant is in a dormant stage. You may dry the roots whole by placing on a screen in a warm airy place, or chop them to hasten the process.

LEGENDARY CURES: Dandelion has a particularly beneficial effect on the liver and is a superior blood cleanser and detoxifier. A European health spa, noted for its eminent physician and cures of all liver complaints, regularly serves Dandelion greens as well as a conventional salad to all patients. The record this man has achieved in his field is quite remarkable and can be attributed, in large part, to the Dandelion's potent powers.

TRADITIONAL USE - INTERNALLY: Authoritative herbologists recommend that diabetics eat up to 10 fresh Dandelion stems daily, gathered when the plant is in bloom. This same treatment brings surprising benefits to the constantly tired and exhausted who never seem to have the energy to do their daily tasks. For chronic inflammation of the liver, 5 or 6 stems per day bring quick relief. The pains of gout, rheumatism and swollen glands disappear when the fresh stems are chewed for a period of time and jaundice and disorders of the spleen yield to the Dandelion also. Note: The stems must be taken for two weeks to a month before evaluating their effect.

The Dandelion root, taken raw or as a tea, contains elements which stimulate the production of the gastric juices and which cleanse the blood and detoxify the entire system, as well as aiding in normalizing the metabolic processes. The root is also a mild diuretic.

PREPARING DANDELION ROOT TEA: Chop finely and soak 2 heaping tablespoons dried Dandelion root, or 1 tablespoon fresh, overnight in about 2 cups of cold water. Bring the mixture to a boil the following day, strain out the residue and sip 30 minutes before breakfast and 30 minutes after breakfast.

PREPARING DANDELION HONEY: Take four heaping handfuls of Dandelion blossoms and immerse in a quart of cold water. Bring slowly to the boiling point. Remove from heat, cover and let stand overnight. The following day, strain through cheesecloth, pressing and squeezing the flowers. Add 2 pounds of sugar and half a lemon, sliced. Simmer uncovered on a very low heat to retain the vitamins. Allow the syrup to simmer until it has cooked down to about half its former volume. The consistency should be about the same as honey. Pour into a sterile glass jar and enjoy on bread, toast, rolls or muffins. Store under refrigeration.

DANDELION AS A SALAD ADDITION: Gather fresh young roots and new leaves in the early spring. Chop and add to any green salad. The young root is crisp and tastes a bit like water chestnuts. The taste of the new leaves is like endive.

DANDELION STEMS: Cut stems from the fresh plant with scissors and snip off the leaves and blossoms. Wash in cold water, chew well and eat 5 to 10 stems daily.

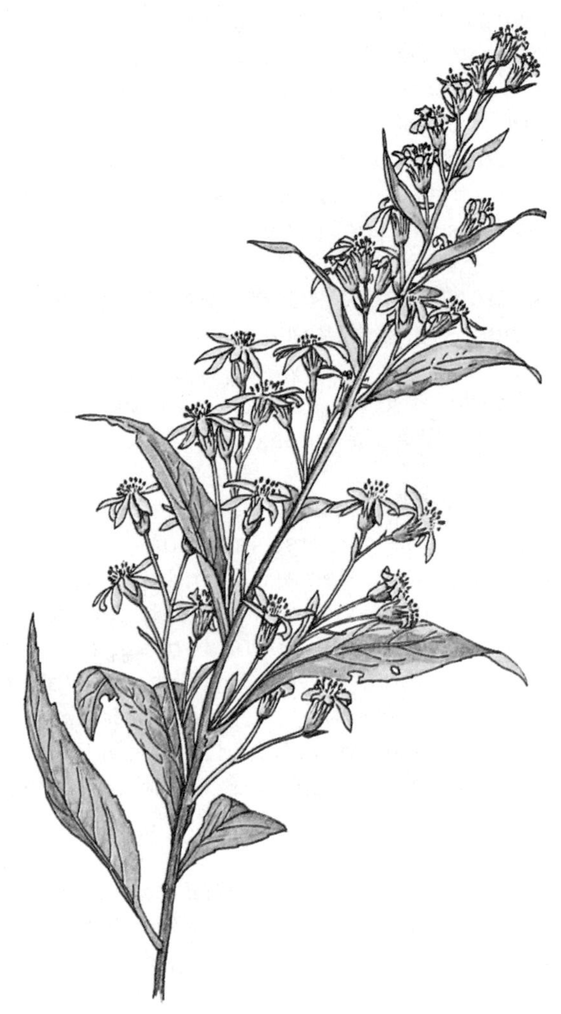

Golden Rod

Solidago virgaurea

Chapter 14
GOLDENROD
(Solidago virgaurea)

Bladder Infections	*Kidney Complaints*	*Shock*
Breath (shortness of)	*Kidneys (cirrhosis)*	*Sweats (cold)*
Emotional Stress	*Kidneys (stones)*	*Wounds*
Intestinal Bleeding	*Kidneys (failure)*	*(promotes healing)*

PAST HISTORY: If you think Golden Rod is good for nothing and only makes you sneeze, you're in for a surprise. It's botanical name comes from the Latin *solidare* and the plant is known as a vulnerary, one that heals wounds and 'makes whole.' Golden Rod has been known and used medicinally since ancient times. The tall rods of glowing gold flowers decorate the plains and woodlands of many countries.

In the first half of the 14th century, the Saracens refused to go into battle without a supply of Golden Rod. This was the favored treatment for wounds and the Crusaders brought the healing knowledge back with them. The early American Indians employed Golden Rod in many remedies and the colonists learned from them. Even cattle love Golden Rod and seek it out in their pastures where it grows freely all over the world.

DESCRIPTION & GROWING REQUIREMENTS: Golden Rod grows to a height of 2 to 3 feet and its slender stem has alternating leaves of a clear green. The stem branches out with many flowering stalks near the top of the central stem. The golden yellow flowers are shaped like tiny stars and Golden Rod can be found in pastures, woods, hillsides and ditches.

Golden Rod makes a pretty addition to the herb garden as a background plant, if no one in the household suffers from seasonal 'hay fever,' and can be dug out and brought home. It transplants easily and is not particular as to soil, but does require adequate moisture.

HOW TO HARVEST & STORE: The flower stalks of Golden Rod may be gathered from mid-summer to fall, July through September, in most areas of the country. Select only the most perfect flowers and cut the whole stem with scissors. Pick off any blemished parts. Tie loosely together in small bunches and hang upside down in a warm airy place to dry.

LEGENDARY CURES: An old herbal written in 1788 tells of a young boy of ten suffering most grievously with a kidney complaint. After drinking Golden Rod tea for several months, it is recorded that the child passed fifteen large stones weighing over 1 ounce, fifty stones over the size of a pea and vast quantities of gravel. Presumably, he made a full recovery.

A very famous Swiss herbalist writes of a 45-year old man by the name of Herman G. who had such a severe kidney condition that one kidney had been surgically removed and the other worked poorly. The herbologist recommended treatment with equal parts of Golden Rod, Cleavers (see Chapter 8) and Yellow Dead Nettle (see Chapter 34). The man was directed to sip 3 to 4 cups of this tea daily. After just two weeks, the cleansing properties of the herbs were effective and Mr. G.'s remaining kidney functioned normally again.

Other writings record the case of Mrs. K., a woman in her fifties suffering from cirrhosis of the kidneys and near renal failure. The poor lady was on a dialysis machine weekly. She was in such a sad state that any activity, even climbing stairs, made her break out into a cold sweat and she became so short of breath that she had to fight for air. I am happy to be able to tell you that the same combination of Golden Rod, Cleavers, and Dead Nettle made into a tea helped Mrs. K. so much that three weeks later she was much improved and able to do her work around the house again for the first time in many years.

TRADITIONAL USE — INTERNALLY: As you can tell from the stories above, Golden Rod is a very potent and effective remedy for all kidney complaints. Bleeding of the intestines and bladder infections yield to Golden Rod and even complete renal failure has been reversed in some cases.

It should be pointed out that the kidneys are overworked when strong emotions are afflicting us, such as a death of a beloved family member or the physical and emotional shock of a severe accident; even the end of a love affair can trigger strong emotions. Golden Rod is invaluable in all cases of emotional shock and stress and comforts and calms, as well as stimulating and cleansing the kidneys.

The Swiss, noted for their natural healing practices, prepare and use a vulnerary tonic called *Faltrank* which employs Golden Rod as a prime ingredient. Even today, this remedy may be easily purchased in local apothecary shops.

PREPARING GOLDEN ROD TEA: Pour 2 cups of boiling water over 2 heaping teaspoons of fresh Golden Rod flowers or 1 heaping teaspoon of dried, cover and steep for 3 to 5 minutes. Strain and sip.

PREPARING GOLDEN ROD COMBINATION TEA: Mix equal parts of Golden Rod, Cleavers and Yellow (or White) Dead Nettles and prepare as directed above. Note: Fresh herbs are recommended in this combination tea.

PREPARING A NATURAL DYE: The leaves and flowers of Golden Rod yield a yellow dye. Gather quantities of the fresh stalks and strip off the leaves and flowers. Immerse in cold water and bring to a boil. Simmer until the infusion is reduced by half. Strain.

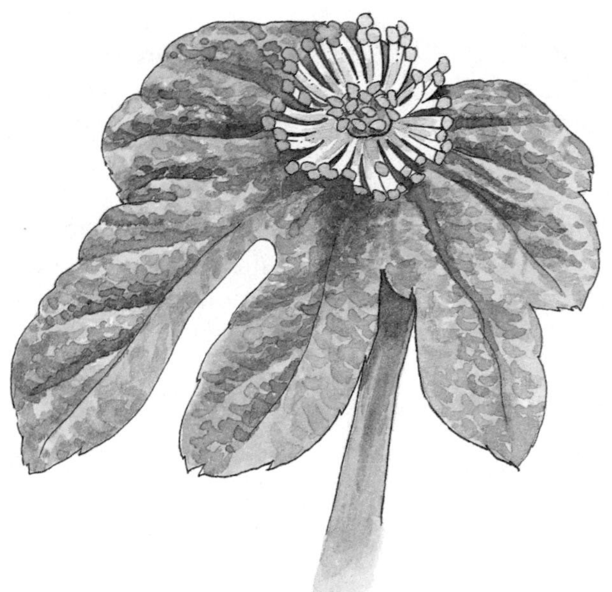

Golden Seal

Hydrastis canadensis

Chapter 15
GOLDEN SEAL
(Hydrastis canadensis)

Appetite (weak)
Bladder Problems
Blood (purifier)
Bronchitis
Colon (inflamed)
Constipation
Digestive Problems
Dyspepsia
Eyes (infected)
Gastric Catarrh
Glandular Aid
Hemorrhoids
Hormonal Stimulant
Infections
Intestinal Tract
Liver Complaints
Mouth (ulcerated)
Mucous Membranes
Nausea
Pitting/Scarring
Poisons (neutralizer)
Rectum (inflamed)
Skin Cleanser
Sweats (night)
Throat (infected)
Tonic
Vomiting

PAST HISTORY: Golden Seal was officially listed in the U.S. Pharmacopeia in 1831 and dropped from this volume in 1936 after being in and out several times during the intervening years. It was introduced in England around 1760. Golden Seal appears in the writings of a Dr. Benjamin Barton in 1798.

Golden Seal was another favorite of the American Indians who used it as a remedy, a dye for clothing and as a face-paint. The root yields a rich gold dye which permeates everything it touches. In the 1800s, an Indian folk healer called Golden Seal one of the "kings of diseases of the mucous membrane unsurpassed by any other known remedy."

DESCRIPTION & GROWING REQUIREMENTS: If you want to grow Golden Seal in your backyard herb garden, you are probably out of luck. Although it transplants well at just about any time of the year, it is very difficult to start Golden Seal from seed and just about impossible to secure as a young plant for transplanting. Fortunately, dried Golden Seal root is readily available.

This perennial is about 6 inches tall and usually bears two rather unattractive wrinkly dark-green hairy leaves. The flowers are small and solitary with greenish-white sepals and appear in April only to fall away immediately after blooming. The fruit of Golden Seal consists of small crimson berries with one or two hard black seeds and ripens in July.

Golden Seal once grew abundantly in the U.S., but was such a valuable addition to the medicine bag that it is rarely found in the wild state any longer. Golden Seal is commercially grown on plantations and the root is harvested after two years growth for sale in herb shops.

LEGENDARY CURES: Golden Seal was commonly used in days of old against dyspepsia, gastric catarrh, to stimulate a weak appetite and in liver troubles. It formed the base of the legendary spring tonics of yesteryear and early physicians recommended Golden Seal 'be snuffed up the nostrils where it causeth great sneezing and the relief of nasal catarrh.'

Bathing the face and other affected areas with an infusion of Golden Seal was believed to prevent the pitting and scarring caused by 'the small pox.'

TRADITIONAL USE — INTERNALLY: Golden Seal is considered a most valuable healing agent in any digestive disorder and exerts a strong action on the mucous membranes everywhere in the body. This potent herb acts to cleanse the bloodstream, helps regulate the liver and has a natural antibiotic effect which stops infections and neutralizes poisons.

It has proven useful in chronic inflammation of the colon and rectum and has been used for hemorrhoids with excellent results. As a tonic, Golden Seal conquers the most stubborn case of long-standing constipation and is a very efficient remedy for nausea and vomiting. Golden seal tea, taken at bedtime, is said to prevent and cure 'night sweats.'

Many respected herbalists recommend Golden Seal to boost the functions of the glandular systems and to stimulate hormonal production. It is a valuable healing agent for bronchial and throat infections, intestinal and bladder conditions.

TRADITIONAL USE — EXTERNALLY: An ulcerated mouth may be soothed and healed by swishing around an infusion of Golden Seal several times a day and the infusion is also an excellent cleanser for the skin. The American Indians used a weak solution of Golden Seal as a treatment for eye infections.

PREPARING GOLDEN SEAL TEA: Golden Seal is used very

sparingly. Steep 1 teaspoon dried Golden Seal root in one cup of boiling water for 3 minutes. Strain and sip. You may sweeten with a little honey, if desired, as the taste is somewhat bitter.
Note: Golden Seal should not be used by pregnant women.

USING GOLDEN SEAL AS A POTENTIATING AGENT: Golden Seal is a valuable addition to any mixture of herbs. Adding 1 teaspoon dried Golden Seal root to approximately 1/2 cup of any blend of herbs will proportionately increase the action of the blend.

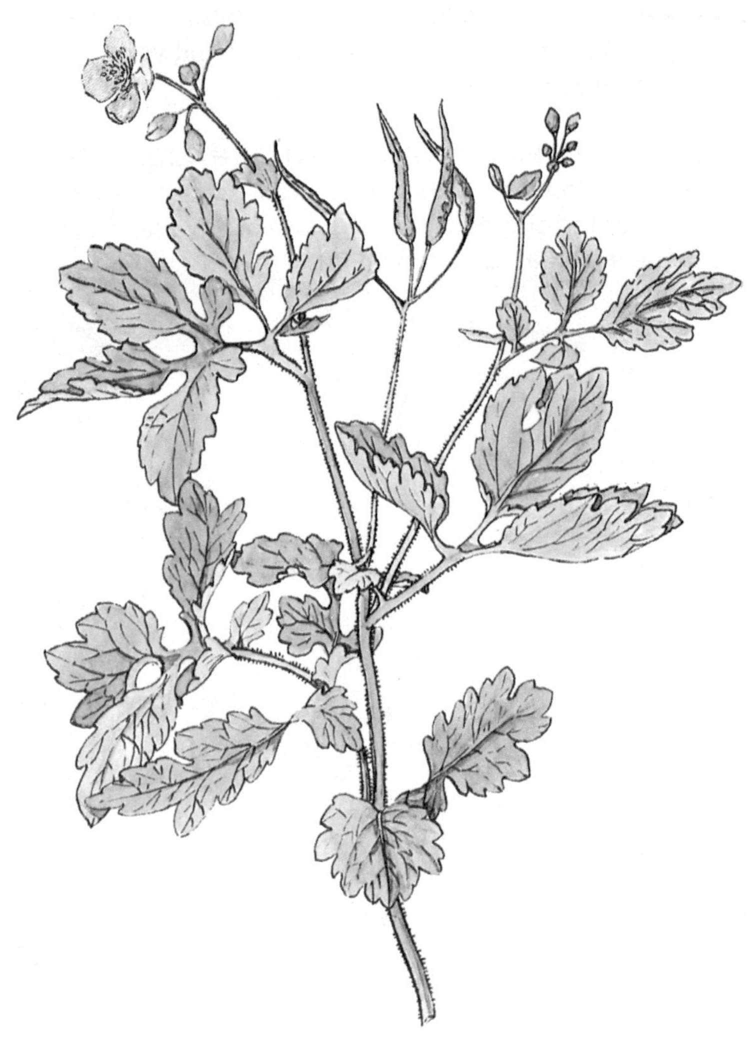

Greater Celadine

Chelidonium majus

Chapter 16
GREATER CELADINE
(Chelidonium majus)

Blood (purifier)
Cancer (skin)
Cataracts
Corns
Ears (ringing in)
Eye-Strain
Gall Bladder
Facial Hair
Hemorrhoids
Herpes Simplex
Jaundice
Kidney Disorders
Leukemia
Liver Complaints
Metabolic Aid
Ringworm
Urination (painful)
Vision Defects
Warts

PAST HISTORY: The Greater Celadine is the true medicinal plant and has nothing in common with the Lesser Celadine, except that the flowers are the same color. Its botannical name comes from *chelidon*, Greek for swallow, so named by Pliny because the Celadine comes into flower when the swallows arrive in the spring and fades as they continue their migration.

As long ago as the 14th century, Celadine was used to strengthen and cleanse the blood. Apothecaries recommended Celadine to "superstifle the jaundice," because of its bright yellow-orange color and the fresh juice was expressed and used in open wounds where it was said to effect an immediate cure.

Celadine was used as a drug plant in the Middle Ages and it was believed the juice dropped into the eye would remove cataracts. An old herbal states, "The juice of the herbe is good to sharpen the sight, for it cleanseth and consumeth away slimie things that cleave about the ball of the eye and hinder the sight and especially being boiled with honey in a brasen vessell, as Dioscorides teacheth."

DESCRIPTION & GROWING REQUIREMENTS: The Greater Celadine is a herbaceous perennial and attains a height from 1-1/2 to 3 feet. Its stem is slender, much branched and slightly hairy with deeply divided leaves resembling those of the mighty oak. Celadine flowers from early spring well into autumn and grows wild in the woods by walls and fences and prefers to face south. The entire plant contains a bright yellow-orange juice which has a powerful odor and rather unpleasant taste.

Celadine is extremely hardy and tolerates both drought and cold. The plant may be found fresh and growing even under a snowy blanket in some climates.

HOW TO HARVEST & STORE: Gather the entire plant when it is in strong flower, usually May through July, and tie into small bundles. Hang the bundles upside down in a warm airy place to dry. Be sure to leave an adequate number of plants to allow it to reseed itself, or gather the seeds themselves for your own garden. The Celadine blossoms are succeeded by long pods containing blackish seeds. The fresh juice is valuable and the herb can provide this juice throughout the year.

LEGENDARY CURES: The tale is told of a farmer's wife who had an ugly reddish protrusion almost half an inch long growing on her lower eyelid. Needing new eyeglasses, the woman went to an ophthalmologist to have her prescription checked and he was horrified by this disfiguring growth. The woman protested that she had had it for almost ten years and it gave her no pain. However, the doctor insisted she go in for a biopsy and the diagnosis was cancer.

The woman was very frightened and immediately began the series of x-ray treatments her physician scheduled for her. A short while later, she ran across an herbalist of her acquaintance who recommended she use the fresh juice of Celadine on the growth. The herbalist supplied the afflicted woman with a potted plant so that she might always have the fresh juice available.

Following the herbalist's recommendations, the woman gently washed a fresh Celadine leaf and crushed the stem of the leaf between her wet thumb and fingers, dabbing the expessed juice on the growth 5 or 6 times daily. Bit by bit, the growth slowly lessened and finally disappeared altogether after some months of this treatment.

When the woman went back to her eye specialist, he was positively dumbfounded that the growth was completely gone and asked her what she had done. She told him she had continued with her monthly x-ray treatments and also used the fresh juice of the Celadine herb. He told her that it is a well-known fact that the x-ray treatments alone cannot shrink and destroy a growth and, indeed, almost always damage surrounding healthy tissue and bone. She confided to him that it was very difficult for her to see the other patients as they came in for their x-ray treatments with flesh and tissue eaten away by cancer to the very bone. She said if it had not been for the hope and faith instilled in her by her herbalist friend, she would have been in despair.

This story surely illustrates the wisdom of the early apothecaries and herbalists who commonly employed the fresh juice of the Greater Celadine to remove and destroy warts, corns, and even ringworm. Celadine is still employed in the U.S.S.R. today where it is said to have been proven effective against some forms of cancer.

To illustrate the power of Celadine in conditions of the eye, I want to remark on a priest of my acquaintance in Austria who successfully used a course of treatment with fresh Celadine to so improve his eyesight that he was able to discard his eyeglasses. The priest's faithful dog actually sat up and begged for Celadine juice after the priest once patted the juice on the animal's eyelids. It seems animals instinctively know what we have to learn.

TRADITIONAL USE - INTERNALLY: Celadine, especially the fresh juice, is a good healer for serious disorders of the liver. Celadine not only cleanses the liver, but also the blood and assists in normalizing a metabolic imbalance as well.

Kidney, liver and gall bladder problems often yield to Celadine. For these problems, the entire fresh plant, gently washed in cold running water, should be put in the juice extractor still wet. The expressed juice is then diluted with twice as much lukewarm water and sipped throughout the day. As a remedy against jaundice, Celadine wine is helpful.

A chronic ringing in the ears, the burning itching discomfort of hemorrhoids and an occasional bout of painful urination yield to Celadine. In these cases, 2 to 3 cups of Celadine tea are sipped during the day.

With its purifying and stimulating properties for the blood, some modern authorities even recommend Celadine against leukemia. A Celadine tea, with Stinging Nettle (see Chapter 28) and Elder shoots is prepared and it is said at least two quarts daily must be drunk over a period of many months for the blend to be effective against this horrendous condition.

TRADITIONAL USE - EXTERNALLY: The traditional herbalist and naturopath employs fresh Celadine juice against cancerous skin disorders, corns and warts. This potent liquid has even proven valuable against herpes simplex lesions.

As medieval herbalists prophesized, Celadine juice may cause cataracts and spots on the cornea of the eye to gradually fade and disappear. Some vision defects and eye-strain yield to Celadine juice also. The juice is extracted from a fresh leaf as outlined above and applied to the outer eyelid gently with the fingertips, but must not be dropped directly into the eye as early herbalists directed. Users report it is as if a veil has been removed and the eyes feel miraculously refreshed.

Some kidney disorders result in an abnormal growth of hair on the face and extremities. Extracted fresh Celadine juice may be patted on the affected areas and allowed to dry for a few hours. Wash off gently with a mild soap and apply either Calendula ointment (see Chapter 5), Chamomile oil (see Chapter 7), or St. John's Wort oil (see Chapter 29). The Celadine juice acts to overdry the skin and the additional moisturizing treatment is of immense benefit in keeping the skin soft and healthy. Horsetail sitz baths (see Chapter 18) and Stinging Nettle tea (see Chapter 28) are also useful aids in stimulating sluggish kidneys and benefit this condition as well.

HOW TO PREPARE CELADINE TEA: Pour 1 pint of freshly boiled water over 2 level teaspoons of Celadine parts. Strain and sip. This is a particularly bitter brew and you may wish to add a little honey to make it more palatable.

HOW TO PREPARE FRESH CELADINE JUICE: Snip the stalk of the entire plant comprising stems, leaves and flowers. Wash gently in cold running water. Don't be dismayed if the parts separate from one another. Place the plant parts still wet in the juice extractor. Note: The fresh juice will remain potent at least six months under refrigeration.

PREPARING CELADINE WINE: Crush an ounce of Celadine parts, fresh or dried and including the root. Place in a quart of dry white wine for 2 hours. Strain through cheesecloth, squeezing the herb parts well with your hands and sip.

CELADINE TINCTURE: In addition to using the fresh juice topically as directed in the text against cataracts and various vision problems, a homeopathic tincture of Celadine taken internally may potentiate the external treatment. The usual recommendation is 10 to 15 drops of Celadine tincture diluted in a cup of water taken two or three times daily. A good herbal shop should be able to provide you with a homeopathic tincture of Celadine.

Chapter 17
HEART WINE
Parsley Honey Wine for the Heart

PAST HISTORY: Over 800 years ago, a holy woman of God wrote down herbal prescriptions that she claimed came to her in visions from the Lord. The Abbess Hildegard von Bingen (1098-1179), now known as Saint Hildegard, was blessed with divine visitations in which certain cures were revealed unto her. Pope Eugen III investigated the Abbess, substantiated her visions, and she was subsequently acknowledged by the Church. This revered holy healer from the past committed her recipes to paper and they have come down to us across the ages in the form of a booklet entitled *God Heals*. This booklet was written by Dr. Hertzka, a General Practitioner in Constance, Lake Constance, Germany.

Dr. Hertzka himself uses the greatest of St. Hildegard's cures, Parsley-Honey Wine for the Heart, in his practice, with great success. He says, "When your heart troubles you, take one, two or even three or more tablespoons of this wine every day. All pains in the heart will disappear as if blown away. You need not be anxious or afraid, because it cannot do any harm. Not only for a slight pain in the heart, but also for cardiac weakness and real heart trouble, this Parsley-Honey Wine will do you a great service, perhaps even bring about a recovery."

LEGENDARY CURES: The files of a renowned European herbalist contain the following letter from a man who is a strong believer in this wonderful remedy. He writes: "I want to tell you that I have prepared the wine and I have obtained the most amazing results. Ten years ago I was operated on and told that I have a weak heart and would always have pain. The doctors said nothing could be done about it and I would just have to accept it. But thanks to this miraculous wine, all my complaints have vanished. After taking this Parsley-Honey Wine for just two months, I don't feel weak anymore!"

TRADITIONAL USE - INTERNALLY: Down through the centuries, St. Hildegard's heavenly remedy has been used with great success against various disorders of the heart, including angina pectoris, pains in the heart of unknown origin and cardiac weaknesses. This potent prescription is reputed to soothe the palpitations of an anxious heart caused by over-excitement and stress as well.

HOW TO PREPARE PARSLEY—HONEY WINE: You will need to have ready a very clean glass bottle which has been sterilized with alcohol. To prepare the wine, add ten fresh parsley stems with the curly leaves attached and two tablespoons of a good quality wine vinegar to one litre (slightly more than one quart) of pure wine (red or white) and simmer for 10 minutes on low heat. Because this mixture foams, use a deep pan. Slowly add 8 ounces of pure honey, stir to dissolve, bring back to simmering temperature, and simmer for an additional 4 minutes. Strain and pour hot into the prepared bottle, using a funnel if necessary. Cork tightly and allow to cool.

It is very important that you prepare the wine in exactly the manner outlined above. The wine, vinegar and parsley must be simmered for 10 minutes before adding the honey and the mixture must again reach simmering temperature and be allowed to simmer for an additional 4 minutes before bottling.

Note: The sediment which forms at the bottom of the bottle over time is not harmful and may be ingested.

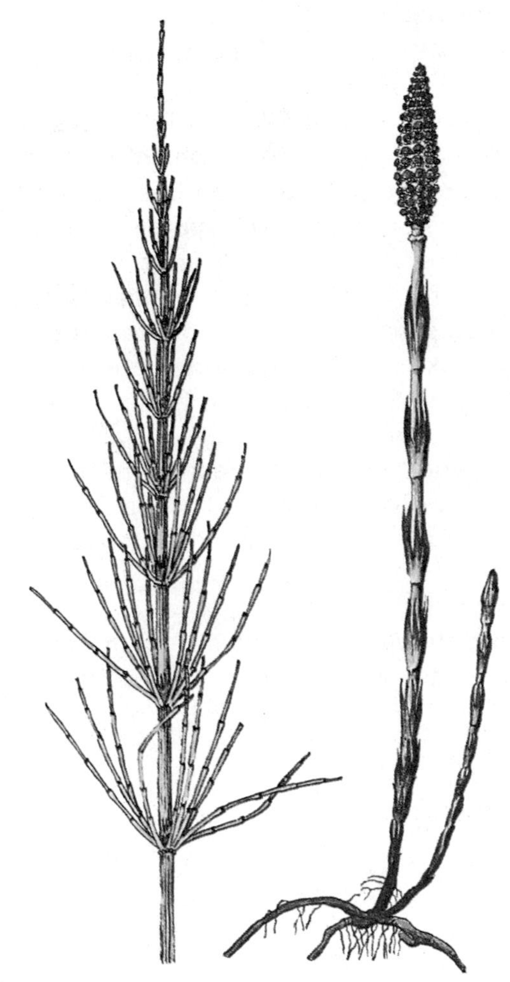

Horsetail

Equisetum arvense

Chapter 18
HORSETAIL
(Equisetum arvense)

Arteriosclerosis
Arthritis
Barber's Itch
Bedwetting
Bladder
Blood (purifier)
Bony Projections
Bronchitis
Bursitis
Cancer (colorectal)
Depression
Disc Lesions
Diuretic
Energy (lack of)
Gall Bladder
Gout
Gums (bleeding)
Hallucinations
Heart (congested)
Hemorrhage
Hemorrhoids
Herpes Simplex
Kidneys
Kidneys (stones)
Liver
Lungs
Mouth/Palate (inflamed)
Muscles (stiff)
Neck (stiff)
Nervous System
Pelvis (inflamed)
Plantar Warts
Pericardium (fluid in)
Pleura (fluid in)
Pylitis
Rage (uncontrolled)
Rheumatism
Skin Rashes
Stomach
Throat (inflamed)
Tonsillitis
Tuberculosis (early)
Urine (suppressed)
Uterus
Vaginal Discharge
Visual Defects
Wounds (supperating)

PAST HISTORY: Just one look at the peculiar configuration of this plant explains how it got its name. Horsetail's botanical name *Equisetum* comes from the Latin words *equus,* horse, and *seta,* bristle. Other common names include Bottle Brush, Shave Grass, Dutch Rushes and Pewterwort and all are indicative of either its appearance or its early uses.

The stems of the Horsetail contain a quantity of silica and were imported from Holland in ages past for use in polishing metal and were often used by kitchen maids of great houses to scour the pewter dishes of the gentry clean. Fine cabinetmakers smoothed and polished their work with Horsetail and dairymaids scoured their milk pails with Horsetail.

Several species of Horsetail have been used medicinally since the early Romans and medieval herbalists recommended Horsetail for consumption, dysentery and praised its healing properties. One surviving manuscript states, "It will heal sinews, though they be cut in sunder."

Master herbalist Culpepper has this to say of Horsetail: "It is very powerful to stop bleeding, either inward or outward. It also heals inward ulcers and solders together the tops of green wounds and cures all ruptures in children. The decoction taken in wine helps stones and the tea strengthens the intestines and is effectual in a cough. The juice is of service in inflammations and breakings-out of the skin."

DESCRIPTION & GROWING REQUIREMENTS: Horsetail can be found growing wild in fields, wet meadows and railway embankments. It is often found growing in hard clay soil and these stands are said to be more valuable medicinally as they draw nutrients from the clay itself. Horsetail has no leaves on its branches, seldom attains a height over three feet and resembles a little brown pine tree.

An old wive's tale says that the presence of Horsetail indicates water underground and wells were often dug on the strength of the Horsetail growing in the area.

HOW TO HARVEST & STORE: In early spring, you will find the fertile single stem of Horsetail culminating in a cat tail, but only the barren stems are of use medicinally. After the fruiting stems have died down, the barren stems arise with their many branches and then is the time to harvest. Cut off the stems just above the root and bring home your prize.

The fresh herb is most potent, but Horsetail may be dried for later use by placing it on a screen in a warm dry place.

LEGENDARY CURES: A respected German herbalist tells of a hard working farmer in his late 40s who was all but incapacitated by a hard growth (possibly a plantar wart) on the sole of one foot. This growth was so painful that he had difficulty walking and had been hospitalized without finding relief. A simple Horsetail poultice first softened and then dissolved the growth within just a few days and the grateful farmer was once again able to work his fields without suffering the agonizing pain that had been with him so long.

This same herbalist has discovered that many times the terrible pain of a disc lesion which causes such suffering may actually be caused by subsequent kidney involvement. One woman who had been under treatment for over three years awoke every morning with her shoulder and neck muscles locked and so stiff she was unable to get out of bed without pulling herself up by grasping a bar her husband fixed over their bed. Just one sitz bath with potent Horsetail quite removed her stiffness and pain and the grateful woman termed it a miracle indeed. Another women under medical treatment for a chronic stiff neck got the same miraculous relief after only 10 minutes in a Horsetail sitz bath.

The underlying theory proven correct in these cases shows that a kidney disorder travels upward along the spinal column and creates pressure on sensitive nerve endings where it causes such pain and stiffness. It was the Horsetail's action on the kidneys which relieved and healed.

TRADITIONAL USE - INTERNALLY: As a natural diuretic, Horsetail is very valuable in all cases of abnormal water retention in the pericardium, pleura, bladder and kidney disorders. The tea, taken for kidney or bladder stones, soon results in a comfortable passing of copious quantities of urine along with the gravel and stones themselves. The treatment involves sipping warm Horsetail tea while holding back the urine as long as possible. A hot Horsetail sitz bath along with the tea is a vital part of this remedy.

When no other diuretic works, from 5 to 6 cups of Horsetail tea should be taken daily for up to a week, or until relief is gained. During this period, no other herb teas should be taken. Experience shows the ingestor will soon pass the unhealthy dark urine easily.

This homely herb is of immense benefit against the common aches and pains of the aged. A cup of Horsetail tea taken daily will eliminate the pain of rheumatism, gout, nerves and arthritis and should be enjoyed all year around. Some authorities believe its action is so strong that it can actually prevent the onset of these conditions if taken regularly. Horsetail tea, with the addition of Speedwell (see Chapter 27), may help prevent hardening of the arteries (arteriosclerosis) as well.

Horsetail is considered extremely valuable for its blood clotting effects and is a specific for hemorrhages of all kinds. It assists in stopping bleeding of the lungs with spitting (or vomiting) of blood, bleeding of the uterus and stomach, and a strong tea of 2 to 3 heaping teaspoons per cup is recommended. Horsetail tea is considered a great remedy for chronic bronchitis and helps heal the lungs, even in cases of tuberculosis. It conquers weakness when taken regularly.

Horsetail tea with St. John's Wort (see Chapter 29) relieves bedwetting when 2 cups daily are taken and no liquid is ingested with the evening meal.

Recent research conducted in Austria by an eminent biologist indicates Horsetail tea may be a cancer prophylactic when taken over a very long period of time. The growth of tumors and polyps (in the abdomen or anus) is slowed and inhibited and they eventually disappear, probably because of the strong blood cleansing action of the silicic acid contained in this plant.

Because kidney disorders are often manifested in depression, hallucination, and physical rage, many of these unhappy people have been misdiagnosed and put away by well meaning family. It has been said that many who would otherwise have ended up in a mental home have come to their senses in time by drinking a cup of Horsetail tea mornings and evenings along with Yarrow tea (see Chapter 33) and Stinging Nettle tea (see Chapter 28). A Horsetail sitz bath is an important adjunct to this treatment.

TRADITIONAL USE - EXTERNALLY: A Horsetail sitz bath, as hot as is comfortable, is recommended for the conditions detailed in the text above. For external use *only* as a sitz bath, the Great or River Horsetail (Equisetum maximum) which grows in bogs, on the banks of rivers and has finger-thick stems, is useful in cases of *pylitis* (an inflammation of the pelvis or outlet of the kidney). A case in point involves a woman hospitalized for weeks with this condition. Just one Horsetail sitz bath so relieved the inflammation, she was able to return home and the pylitis has not returned. In addition, a Horsetail sitz bath so stimulates the kidneys, that young mothers who experience visual defects after a hard labor and difficult birth find their vision clearing as the pressure exerted by the kidneys is relieved. A Horsetail sitz bath has been known to clear a chronic vaginal discharge as well.

In fact, for any kidney disorder, a full Horsetail bath or sitz bath is beneficial. Take care to completely immerse the kidney region and relax for at least 20 minutes. Immediately wrap up in a bathrobe and slip into bed under heavy covers. This should induce copious perspiration. After an hour, change to dry night clothes and enjoy the best night's sleep you've had in years.

For cramping and painful bladder distention, the hot steam of a Horsetail decoction can bring relief. The recommended method is to disrobe and wrap up in a thick towel or bathrobe and allow the steam to work into the area for at least 10 minutes. Repeated several times, this method may make the use of a catheter unnecessary.

A Horsetail poultice or compress is of value for cleansing open supperating wounds or ulcers and may even burn away cancer-like growths. These poultices also relieve stomach pain, liver and gall bladder attacks, bursitis and congestion of the heart.

A Horsetail wash or compress is helpful in relieving itchy rashes, even if they are scabbed or festering. A wash or bath is beneficial for cracked and festering wounds of all kinds, abnormal bony projections, old wounds, fistulas, barber's itch and even herpes simplex lesions. For relieving the pain and itch of hemorrhoids or hemorrhoidal polyps, the pulp of Horsetail is applied to the affected area.

Horsetail tea is an excellent gargle for tonsillitis, inflammation of the mucous membranes of the mouth and throat, bleeding gums, and helps heal inflammations of the palate.

HOW TO PREPARE HORSETAIL TEA: Pour 6 ounces of freshly boiled water over 1 heaping teaspoon of the herb. Cover, steep for four minutes, strain and sip hot. You may add a little honey, if you like.

HOW TO PREPARE A HORSETAIL TINCTURE: Loosely fill a glass bottle with fresh Horsetail parts, finely minced. Add pure spirts to cover. Shake daily, and allow the bottle to stand in a warm place for two weeks. Strain, bottle, and cork tightly.

HOW TO PREPARE A HORSETAIL POULTICE: Place two heaping handfuls of Horsetail in a collander over boiling water. Cover tightly to keep in the steam. After the herb parts are soft and hot, wrap in a clean white cloth and apply to the affected part. Double wrap with additional cloth to hold in the heat.

HOW TO PREPARE A HORSETAIL PULP COMPRESS: Wash a quantity of fresh Horsetail under running water. While still wet, crush, and turn onto a clean white cloth. Apply as above.

HOW TO PREPARE A HORSETAIL BATH: Soak a quantity of fresh Horsetail in cold water overnight. The following day, bring the mixture to a boil, strain, and add a suitable amount to either a sitz bath or full bath. Soak for a full 20 minutes in a full bath, making sure the water covers the kidneys. Immediately wrap up warmly and go to bed for one hour. You will perspire freely.

Chapter 19
LADY'S MANTLE
(Alchemilla vulgaris)

Abdomen (Inflamed)
Anemia
Appetite (weak)
Childbirth
Diabetes
Diuretic
Epilepsy
Failure to Thrive
Female Disorders
Fever
Heart Disorders
Heart (strengthener)
Hemorrhage
Hernias
Hot-Flashes
Insect Bites
Insomnia
Menopausal Problems
Menstrual Problems
Miscarriage
Multiple Sclerosis
Muscles (weak)
Muscular Atrophy
Obesity
Ovarian Cysts
Premenstrual Symptoms
Puberty
Reproductive Organs
Skin Irritations
Sores (old)
Tooth (extraction)
Ulcers
Urethral Irritation
Urine (burning)
Uterus (prolapse of)
Vaginal Discharge
Wounds (suppurating)

PAST HISTORY: The botanical name for Lady's Mantle comes from the Arabic *alkemelych* (alchemy) and was bestowed upon it, according to old manuscripts, because of its wonder-working powers. In the Middle Ages, the plant was likened to the Virgin Mary's mantle because the graceful scalloping of the leaves resembled the scalloped edges of a woman's cloak.

Culpepper esteemed Lady's Mantle and wrote: "Lady's Mantle is very proper for inflamed wounds and to stay bleeding, vomitings, fluxes of all sorts, bruises by falls and ruptures." In both the past and present, Lady's Mantle has been termed essentially a 'woman's herb' and is valuable for all manner of 'female complaints.'

DESCRIPTION & GROWING REQUIREMENTS: This graceful little plant likes grassy pastures, woodlands and high mountainous regions. Its kidney-shaped leaves are lobed and it bears small greenish-yellow flowers. At high altitudes, the Silver Lady's Mantle may be found growing happily on limestone and basalt. Both plants offer the same valuable medicinal qualities.

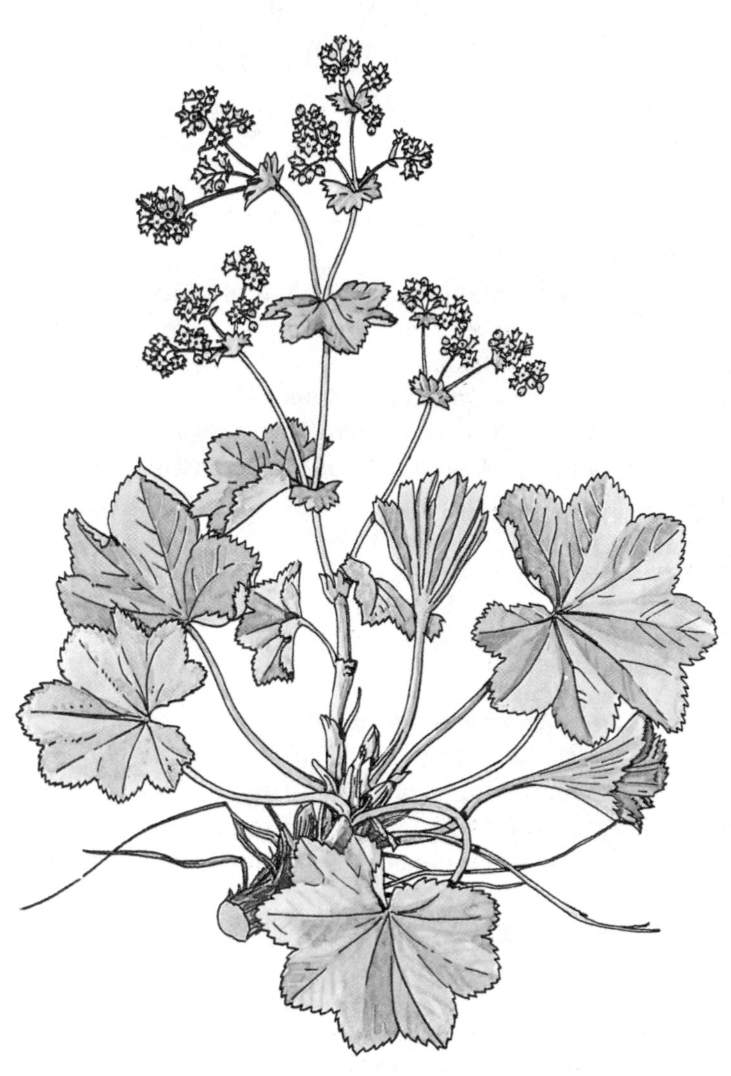

Lady's Mantle
Alchemilla vulgaris

HOW TO HARVEST & STORE: The whole plant is gathered when in flower, usually from April to June, but Lady's Mantle may be found flowering as late as August in some climates. After the flowers have dropped, harvest the leaves by pinching them off.

If you bring home whole plants, tie them into bunches and hang upside down in a warm airy place to dry thoroughly. Dry the leaves separately on a screen to allow air to circulate.

LEGENDARY CURES: For all female complaints and disorders, Lady's Mantle has no equal. A young woman, Mary M., was in much distress because she suffered dreadfully in childbirth. After being delivered of her first child, she hemorrhaged and very nearly died in spite of the doctor's administrations. She learned of the words of a great German herbalist, who said, "Every woman in childbed should drink much of this tea. Some children would still have their mother, some stricken widower his wife, had they but known of Lady's Mantle."

Mary M. began taking an infusion of Lady's Mantle daily over some months and the birth of her second child was perfectly normal, thanks to the strengthening properties of this herb. Lady's Mantle proved once again, as it has for centuries, to strengthen both fetus and uterus. Women who have a history of miscarriages, those who have weak abdominal muscles and any who have reason to suspect a difficult delivery should take Lady's Mantle for its healing and strength-building properties to the female organs, but only after the third month of pregnancy.

TRADITIONAL USE - INTERNALLY: In addition to the uses outlined above, Lady's Mantle is of immense help in the whole range of general female complaints, such as PMS (premenstrual tension), menstrual difficulties of all kinds, ovarian cysts, urethral irritation, vaginal discharges and so on. Lady's Mantle, with Yarrow (see Chapter 33), promotes a comfortable first period for a young girl entering puberty. After menopause, Lady's Mantle eliminates or mitigates hot-flashes and soothes menopausal nervous symptoms as well.

This herb is indeed a 'cure-all' for all female disorders. Used with Shepherd's Purse (see Chapter 26), it aids in cases of prolapse of the uterus and hernias. For these conditions, it is necessary to take four cups of the tea daily, preferably prepared from the fresh herb. A brisk massage of the area with Shepherd's Purse Tincture assists, as does a thrice-weekly sitz bath with Yarrow (see Chapter 33).

The benefits of Lady's Mantle for women have been well expressed by a noted Swiss herbalist, as follows: "With early and prolonged use of this medicinal herb, two-thirds of all operations performed on women would be unnecessary. It heals all inflammations of the abdomen, fever, burning, suppuration, ulcers and hernias."

In spite of the wide range of female disorders Lady's Mantle benefits, it is not for women only. Used with Shepherd's Purse, it relieves and strengthens in cases of muscular atrophy and aids in some currently incurable diseases affecting the muscles, such as multiple sclerosis.

Children who fail to thrive and who have weak musculature also benefit by continual drinking of the tea. Because of its astringent properties, Lady's Mantle is recommended as a cardiac strengthener and is said to restore appetite in anemics of all ages. Diabetics benefit, as do insomniacs and early herbals suggest Lady's Mantle for epileptics as well.

In all cases of overweight and obesity, two to three cups of tea taken daily are said to act both as an appetite depressant and a mild diuretic.

TRADITIONAL USE - EXTERNALLY: A wash of Lady's Mantle cleans and quickly heals festering wounds and old sores which refuse to close. When the wash is massaged gently into the chest, Lady's Mantle is reputed to relieve disorders of the heart muscle. Mild and soothing, this herb, crushed, promotes healing of cuts, stings, insect bites, and open bruises and is particularly useful for children's scrapes and scratches. Used as a rinse after having a tooth extracted, this astringent herb quickly heals the open wound overnight.

HOW TO PREPARE LADY'S MANTLE TEA: Pour 6 ounces of freshly boiled water over one heaping teaspoon of the herb. Cover and steep for three to five minutes. Strain and sweeten with a little honey, if desired.

HOW TO PREPARE A WOUND DRESSING: Gather a quantity of fresh Lady's Mantle. Wash gently and crush well with a rolling pin. Apply to affected parts.

HOW TO PREPARE A WASH OR BATH: For a wash, immerse one handful of the fresh herb in a quart of cold water and allow to soak overnight. The following day, warm slowly to body temperature and use as directed in the text as a wash or rinse. To prepare a full or sitz bath, use three double handfuls of the herb and soak overnight in a gallon of cold water. Warm and add a suitable quantity of the potent liquid to a sitz bath or the entire gallon to a full bath.

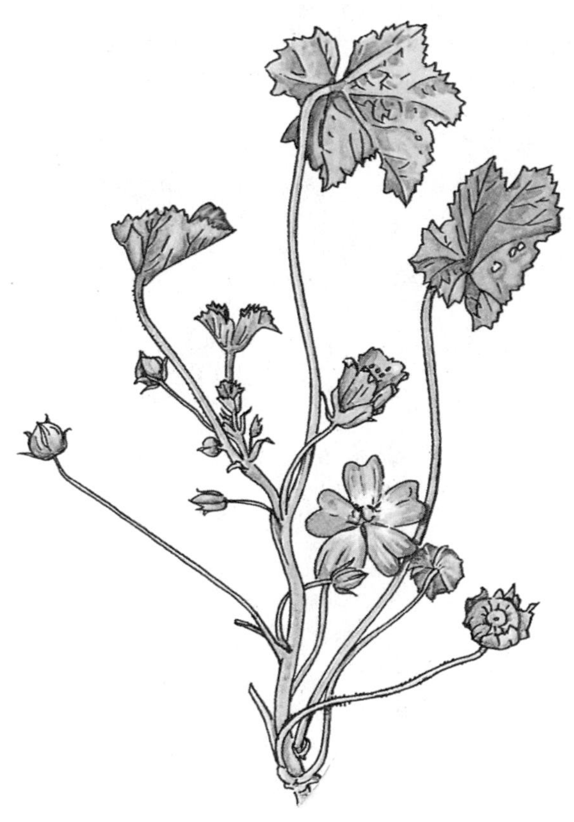

Mallow

Malva vulgaris

Chapter 20
MALLOW
(Malva Vulgaris)

Bedsores	*Digestive Tract*	*Skin Allergies*
Bladder	*Hives*	*Skin Conditions*
Bones (fracture)	*Hoarseness*	*Sprains*
Breath (shortness of)	*Intestines*	*Stomach Upsets*
Bronchitis	*Laryngitis*	*Swellings (abnormal)*
Cancer (larynx)	*Lungs*	*Tear-Ducts (clogged)*
Coughs	*Mouth (inflamed)*	*Throat Disorder*
Cystitis	*Mouth (dry)*	*Throat (dry)*
Emphysema	*Mucous Membranes*	*Tonsillitis*
Extremities (swollen)	*Nasal Passages (dry)*	*Ulcers*
Eyes (strained)	*Phlebitis*	*Voice (loss of)*
Gastritis	*Phlegm (tough)*	*Wounds*

PAST HISTORY: The family of Mallows, of which there are many sub-species, has been esteemed for centuries. The name Malva comes from the Greek, *malake* (soft) and refers to the special properties of the Mallows in softening and healing. In Job 30:4, we find Mallow mentioned as being eaten in time of famine and it is known that most of the Mallows have been used as food through the ages. Charlemagne, A.D. 742-814, directed that Mallow be served at his table. Both the Romans and the Chinese considered Mallow a delicacy. In Syria and Egypt yet today, the Mallows are cultivated and eaten with much pleasure.

In the writings of Dioscorides, a Greek physician of the first century noted as the author of authoritative works on natural medicinals of the day, the virtues of Mallow were upheld. Mallow was so highly regarded, it was used to decorate the graves of special friends. Pliny, the ancient herbalist of such note, said "Whosoever shall take a spoonful of the Mallows shall that day be free from all diseases that mayst come to him."

Today, both French and English apothecaries prepare a paste of Mallow which is emollient and soothing and very valuable in conquering coughs, sore throats and hoarseness. Mallow is one of the prime ingredients of the *Tisane de quatre fleurs*, a particularly pleasant cold remedy still sold in France.

Just in case you're wondering, the marshmallows found in today's supermarkets are no longer made with anything resembling the Mallow plant. They are a gummy mixture of flour, gum, egg-white (albumin), powdered sugar and chemical preservatives. Now, don't you wish you didn't know?

DESCRIPTION & GROWING REQUIREMENTS: The Mallows were popularly cultivated as little as fifty years ago and, though they now thrive wild on walls and pathways, they are almost always found growing where a home once stood. Many varieties take well in home gardens and they are an important addition to any herbal plot as their properties are most potent in the fresh state.

The small leafed Mallow has long slender stems, rounded toothed leaves and bears small pale pink or purplish flowers. Its round fruits are known as 'cheeses,' which country-bred children sometimes eat or play with. Mallow may be grown from seed or cuttings.

HOW TO HARVEST & STORE: The entire plant offers us mucilage (a soothing, coating demulcent) and tannin (an astringent mucous solvent), as does the large leafed Mallow. The flowers, leaves and stems may be harvested spring to fall, usually June through September. In dried form, Mallow still retains a portion of its medicinal qualities, but has lost a great degree of its mucilage. It is best used fresh.

LEGENDARY CURES: The power and potency of the Mallow is amply demonstrated in the history of Henry McD. This unfortunate man had been hospitalized and treated many times in many months for a throat affliction and eventually quite lost his voice. Being unable to speak, his wife spoke for him and finally called on a renowned herbalist, expressing her fears that her beloved husband was actually suffering from cancer of the larynx. She told of her frustration in that the doctors would not tell her anything.

The herbalist advised Mrs. McD. to have her husband gargle frequently with an infusion (tea) of Mallow and to apply a poultice of the tea residue, blended with barley flour, to his throat overnight. This the woman did and was overjoyed to find her husband recovered his voice within two weeks and felt so well he was able to return to work.

An interesting epilogue to this story concerns Henry McD.'s doctor who approves of the medicinal herbs. He was so pleased with the improvement in his patient's condition, he remarked, "That herbalist deserves a gold medal!"

Helena G., on the recommendation of her mother, tried Mallow to soothe a case of chronic cystitis which had caused her great pain for a lengthy period. Ms. G. took a cupful of Mallow tea three times daily after meals and was delighted to find herself free of pain for the first time in many, many months, thanks to the soothing coating effect of the Mallow.

Even externally, Mallow proves quite remarkable against sprains and swellings that refuse to subside. George J., an elderly gentleman, fell and suffered a severe ankle sprain. Before trying the Mallow soak, he had been forced to walk with a cane for over three weeks because his foot became so swollen during the day he could barely hobble along. Mr. J. found relief after just a few good soakings in a Mallow foot bath.

TRADITIONAL USE - INTERNALLY: The Mallow is of benefit in so many conditions, it must be considered one of mankind's most remarkable medicinal plants. For inflammations of all the mucous membranes, including the gastro-intestinal tract, the bladder, the stomach, the intestines and even the mouth, Mallow provides prompt healing relief. Cystitis, gastritis and ulcers succumb to Mallow's properties.

For all the above conditions, a Barley/Mallow soup is made by first cooking the barley and, after cooling to room temperature, blending in finely chopped Mallow leaves.

To prepare Mallow for bronchitis, coughs, hoarseness, tonsillitis, laryngitis and phlegm in the lungs (including emphysema), soak a quantity of Mallow overnight in cold water. Because heat destroys the mucilaginous properties of the herb, Mallow should not be cooked or heated. Warm the infusion the following day slightly and sip two to three cups throughout the day for prompt relief and easier breathing.

Certain European herbalists have recently reported great success in relieving malignant disorders of the larynx with Mallow. For inflammation and severe involvement of the larynx, at least 2-1/2 quarts of a strong infusion of Mallow must be used daily, prepared by using 5 heaping teaspoons of the herb steeped overnight in 2-1/2 quarts of pure cold water. The tea may be warmed slightly for palatability. Four cups should be sipped slowly throughout the day and the balance used for a deep gargle until the whole is used up.

TRADITIONAL USE - EXTERNALLY: A lukewarm Mallow wash soothes skin allergies and the burning and itching of hives. This wash also speeds healing of wounds and skin ulcerations of all kinds. Old sores which refuse to heal will begin to granulate and close overnight after washing with Mallow and applying fresh Plantain leaves (see Chapter 23).

If someone you love suffers from long-standing bedsores, please try washing a fresh Plantain leaf and applying, still wet, on the open wound which has first been soothed with a Mallow wash. The patient should also take Mallow tea during the day. This combination treatment really brings the most amazing results. Swollen feet and hands, even when caused by phlebitis or a bad fracture, benefit from a Mallow soak lasting at least 20 minutes per treatment.

A gargle and rinse with a Mallow infusion used frequently throughout the day often relieves annoying chronic dryness of the mouth, throat and nose and provides a most soothing coating. Mallow is so mild, it is even beneficial as an eye-wash and opens up clogged tear-ducts. A warm compress of Mallow applied in the eye area is as effective as anything I've ever seen for relieving eye-strain and restoring tired eyes to their normal brightness.

PREPARING THE COLD INFUSION OF MALLOW: Soak one heaping teaspoon of the herb overnight in 6 ounces of cold fresh water. You may warm slightly in the morning before drinking the tea or using it as a wash as directed above. Remember, Mallow must *not* be heated, only gently warmed.

PREPARING A MALLOW FOOT OR HAND BATH: Soak two heaping handfuls of Mallow overnight in 2-1/2 quarts of cold water. The following day, warm to lukewarm and immerse the affected part in the solution for at least 20 minutes. The bath may be used three times in all before it loses effectiveness.

PREPARING A MALLOW POULTICE: After making the cold

infusion as directed above, strain off the tea for drinking and save the residue. Warm slightly in a small quantity of water, mix in a bit of barley flour and spread on a piece of clean white cloth. Apply warm.

AN OLD-COUNTRY POULTICE: An old-country recipe for preparing a Mallow poultice directs that the residue from the cold infusion be warmed, heaped on a slice of white bread and then applied directly to the affected part.

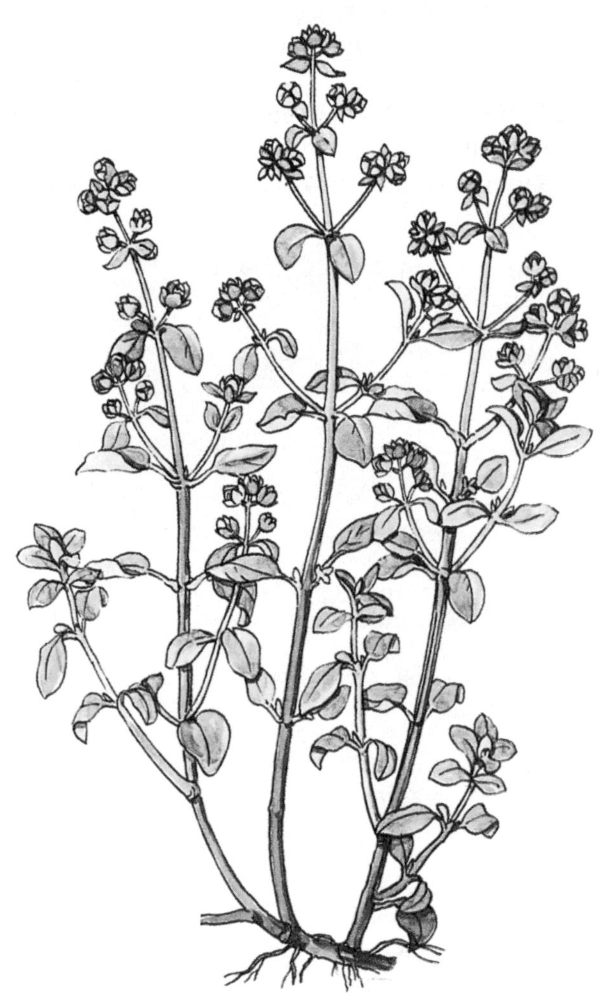

Marjoram

Marjorana hortensis

Chapter 21
MARJORAM
(Marjorana hortensis)

Appetite (weak)
Arthritis
Asthma
Bowels (sluggish)
Bronchial Aid
Colic
Coughs
Depression
Diarrhea
Dizziness
Expectorant
Gastritis
Glands (swollen)
Headaches
Jaundice
Joints (stiff)
Liver Disorders
Menstruation (irregular)
Migraine
Mouth(inflamed)
Muscles (strained)
Nervous System
Nose (stuffy)
Rheumatism
Stomach (nervous)
Toothache
Throat (inflamed)
Varicose Veins

PAST HISTORY: Marjoram's botanical name, 'Origanum marjorana,' comes from two Greek words, *oros* (mountain) and *ganos* (joy) and appears to refer to the joyful look these pretty plants confer to the hills on which they flourish in the wild.

Marjoram has been used for untold centuries for its medicinal qualities. Ancient Greek physicians valued it as an agent for poisons, convulsions and dropsy. The early Greeks believed Marjoram growing on a grave promised happiness to the dear departed and both Greeks and Romans crowned newly married couples with sweet Marjoram to insure the happiness of the union.

This fragrant plant was a favorite 'strewing herb' in medieval England where it was prized as an air freshener. Master Herbalist Parkinson mentions Marjoram in this connection and also wrote, "The swete (translated as 'sweet,' not 'sweat') margerome is used in swete bags, swete powders and swete washing water." At one point in time, the aromatic juices of the herb were used to polish furniture.

Country folk still sometimes use the flowering tops of Marjoram as a dye, but the colors tend to fade quite rapidly. When used on woolens, Marjoram gives a purple tint; on linens, the color is a reddish-brown hue.

Early herbalists used a few drops of Marjoram oil on lint and tucked it into a decayed tooth to stop the hurt. The dried leaves and tops were applied topically to ease the pain of rheumatism, gout and colic. An infusion (tea) was said to bring out 'measles spots' quickly and was recommended to relieve nervous headaches and to give fast relief from pain in dyspeptic complaints, spasms and colic.

DESCRIPTION & GROWING REQUIREMENTS: Sweet Marjoram, the type you will most likely want in your garden, is a perennial which is treated as an annual. This tender herb is a native of Portugal and difficult to winter over in most climates.

Marjoram has a creeping root system and wooly red-brown stems which grow to a height of seven to seventeen inches, crowned with rounded bunches of tiny flowers. Marjoram's leaves are small and elliptical and radially positioned on the branched upright stems. Marjoram likes a light, sandy soil and may be grown from seed. Don't be impatient. Marjoram is slow to germinate.

HOW TO HARVEST & STORE: In olden times, Marjoram cultivated for the apothecary shops was scythed down and the cut plants were beaten with wooden staves to separate the leaves from the stems. This resulted in broken leaves mixed with the debris of the stems. We suggest you cut the stems of the mature, flowering herb (July to September in most climates), and tie in small bunches. Hang the entire herb upside down in a warm, airy place to dry.

LEGENDARY USES: A charming superstition from ages past tells us that fanciful young ladies who wished to know the man they would marry concocted a potion of Marjoram from the following instruction: 'On St. Luke's Day, take ye a sprig of Marjoram, the flowers of Marigold and Thyme. Dry them before a fire and rub them into a powder. Sift through a piece of fine lawn and add a small quantity of virgin honey and vinegar to the herbs. Simmer the potion over a slow fire. Anoint yourself before going to bed, saying these lines thrice: "St. Luke, St. Luke, be kind to me. In dreams let me my true love see."' Legend has it that this magic charm and fragrant anointing assured dreams of the future partner 'that is to be.'

TRADITIONAL USE — INTERNALLY: Marjoram is a well-known and favorite seasoning herb. What you may not know is that Marjoram encourages a weak appetite, stimulates the action of sluggish bowels, relieves all kinds of cramps and soothes stomach upsets by stimulating the necessary gastric secretions which digest our food. A cup of Marjoram tea will often halt diarrhea.

The action of Marjoram is mildly disinfectant and carminative. An infusion of Marjoram (tea) dissolves bronchial mucous and acts as a superior expectorant. This tea is particularly soothing for a sore throat, resulting coughs and even asthma. Marjoram is so mild in action it is suitable for a child suffering colic or abdominal pain from gas. Gastritis often yields to Marjoram and positive experiences have been reported abroad using Marjoram against liver disorders, particularly jaundice.

Marjoram tea is traditionally given in cases of depression, chronic headaches, migraine, dizziness and a 'nervous' stomach. Marjoram acts to invigorate the entire nervous system. A combination of Marjoram and several other herbs (see 'How to Prepare' at the close of the chapter) is a great help in regulating menstruation.

TRADITIONAL USE — EXTERNALLY: As the ancient herbalists discovered, Marjoram helps quiet an aching tooth and, used as a mouth rinse or gargle, assists in healing all inflammations of the mouth and throat.

The warming effect of Marjoram oil used in a gentle massage helps relieve the pain of aching strained muscles, the stiffened joints of the arthritic and rheumatic and even relieves swollen glands and varicose veins. A pillow of Sweet Marjoram placed on the affected part is a useful adjunct to the oil massage.

A stuffy nose may be cleared and drained of tough mucus by sniffing a small quantity of the dried and pulverized herb. Be prepared to sneeze violently.

HOW TO PREPARE A MARJORAM INFUSION (TEA): Pour 6 ounces of freshly boiled water over two teaspoons of the dried herb. Cover and steep for three minutes. Strain and sweeten with a bit of honey, if desired. Sip one to two cups daily as hot as is comfortable.

HOW TO PREPARE MARJORAM COMBO TEA FOR IRREGULAR MENSTRUATION: Blend together 2 tablespoons each of Marjoram, Yarrow, Thyme, Fennel and Hops with 4 tablespoons Valerian and 3 tablespoons Frangula. Pour 6 ounces of freshly boiled water over 2 heaping tablespoon of the herb combination and steep, covered, for three minutes. Take one cupful of the warm tea mornings and evenings for the 10 days preceeding the onset of the menses.

HOW TO PREPARE MARJORAM OIL: Lightly crush a quantity of dried Marjoram and half-fill a clean glass (not plastic) bottle. Add cold-pressed olive oil to the rim. Cork tightly and place the bottle in a warm place for three weeks. Strain off the residue and use the oil as a massage aid.

HOW TO PREPARE A MARJORAM PILLOW: Crush a quantity of the dried herb and fill a small pillow of tightly woven cloth. Apply overnight to painful joints for a comforting night's sleep.

Chapter 22
MISTLETOE
(Viscum album)

Arteriosclerosis
Blood Pressure
Cancer (breast)
Chilblains
Circulatory Stimulant
Dizziness
Diabetes
Ears (ringing in)
Energizer
Epilepsy
Glandular Stimulant
Heartbeat (irregular)
Heart (strengthener)
Hormonal Imbalance
Infertility
Menstruation
Menstrual Cramps
Menopausal Problems
Metabolic Imbalance
Mucous Membranes
Nervous Complaints
Nosebleed
Pancreas
Stroke
Visual Defects

PAST HISTORY: Mistletoe is sometimes called *Herbe de la Croix.* According to an old Christian legend, the Cross was made from Mistletoe and it was for that reason the plant was turned into a parasite which cannot grow without a host tree.

The familiar custom of kissing under the Mistletoe at Christmas may have its roots in a Scandanavian tale of the ancient god, Balder, the mythological god of Peace. Balder was supposedly slain by his enemies with an arrow made of Mistletoe. Balder was restored to life when the other gods and goddesses petitioned on his behalf. The Mistletoe was then given to the goddess of Love for safekeeping and she ordained that everyone passing under it must receive a kiss to show it was a missile of love, not hate.

The Druids revered Mistletoe and, garbed in white robes, gathered it only during a certain phase of the moon, cutting it from the tree with a knife of gold. If the Mistletoe fell to the ground of its own accord, the Druids believed a great misfortune would come upon the land. Druid priests were said to have wrought wonderous cures with Mistletoe sprigs.

In 15th century France, Mistletoe was the remedy of choice against epilepsy and in 1720, Sir John Colbatch wrote a paper entitled *The Treatment of Epilepsy by Mistletoe.* Sir John directed "the powdered leaves of Mistletoe, as much as would lie on a sixpence, be given in Black Cherry water every morning" as a specific for epilepsy. Mistletoe

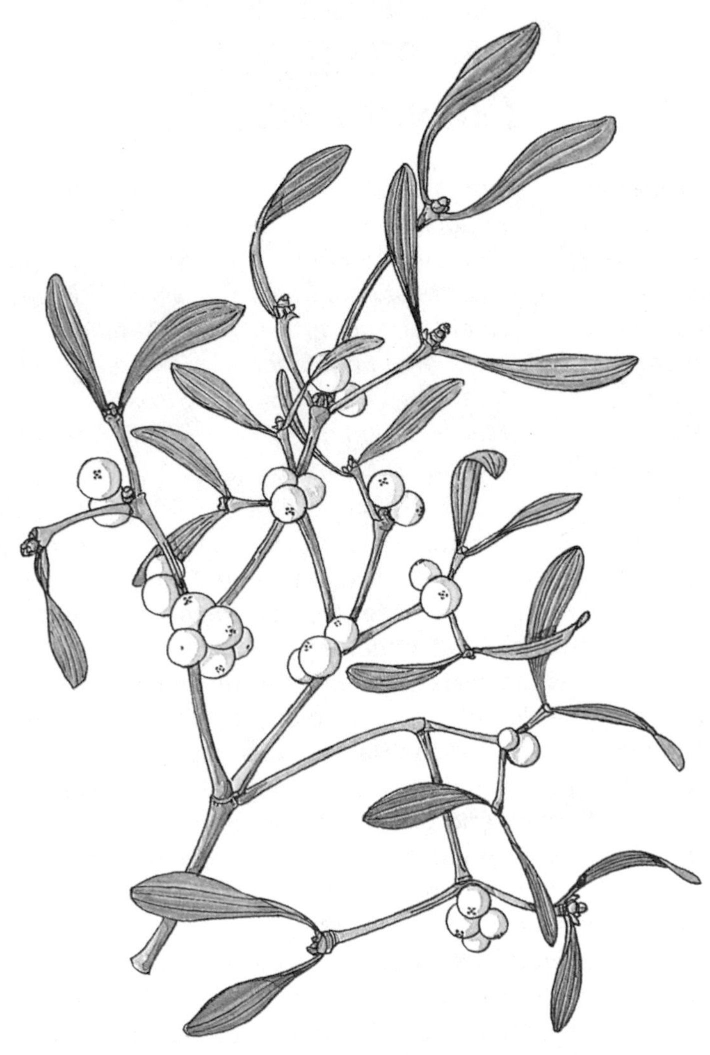

Mistletoe

Viscum album

has long been considered efficacious in treatment of all nervous disorders, including St. Vitus Dance.

DESCRIPTION & GROWING REQUIREMENTS: Everyone is probably familiar with the yellow-green leaves and white berries of the Mistletoe. This parasite grows on deciduous and pine trees, such as oak, poplar, pines, firs and fruit trees. The herbs with the strongest medicinal qualities are found on oak and poplar trees, but those fastened to pines, firs and fruit trees also yield good medicinal properties.

Mistletoe cannot be grown in earth or water, but you can cultivate the plant if you have a suitable tree. Imitate nature by rubbing the berries on the smooth bark of the underside of a branch until it sticks, or make a small cut and insert a few berries. After a few days, the Mistletoe will send out a fine root which finally pierces the bark and embeds itself in the living tree. The Mistletoe will then nourish itself with the juices of the tree.

HOW TO HARVEST & STORE: Gather the leaves and small twigs for drying from October through December and again in March and April. For reasons best known to Mother Nature, the herb has no medicinal qualities during the other months of the year. Remove and discard any berries (or put them aside if planning to make ointment) and spread the leaves and twigs on a screen. Place the screen in a warm dry place. Note: The fresh berries are used *only* in ointment and never taken internally. They are poisonous.

LEGENDARY CURES: If you live in a cold climate and suffer from chilblains (an extreme inflammation of the extremities aggravated by cold), you will be particularly interested to hear of William G. who had chilblains of the nose to the extent that he dreaded going to work every day because of the jokes his co-workers made about the bluish-red coloring of his nose. His wife consulted an herbalist and followed his directions, gathering fresh Mistletoe berries, crushing them into a bit of pure lard and applying the ointment to Mr. G.'s nose overnight. After just a week of this treatment, Mr. G. was delighted to find his painful and embarrassing problem was gone and his nose was the same color as the rest of his face.

Internally, an even more important effect Mistletoe exerts is the normalizing of blood pressure, whether low or high. I remember going into the woods with my aged grandmother one very cold day to cut Mistletoe. A farmwife of her acquaintance, Jenny B., who had five children and a tremendous workload, had all but taken to her bed because her blood pressure was so low it couldn't sustain her energies. Grandmother told Mrs. B. to sip three cups of a cold infusion of Mistletoe daily. Within just a few weeks, Jenny B. came over to Grandmother's house to thank her with all her heart for restoring her quite completely.

Grandmother always said that Mistletoe should be taken regularly for six weeks out of every year to regulate blood pressure, banish dizziness, strengthen a weak heart, stimulate circulation and restore energy. In the fall when Mistletoe is at the height of its powers, she made a quantity of the cold infusion. We were all to take three cups daily for three weeks, then two cups for two weeks and one cup for the final week. (This course of treatment is also of benefit to stroke victims.) After this yearly treatment, it is best to sip a cup of the cold infusion daily with breakfast to keep Mistletoe's powers working constantly.

TRADITIONAL USE - INTERNALLY: In addition to the conditions outlined above, all circulatory problems yield to Mistletoe, including hardening of the arteries (arteriosclerosis), and certain heart conditions (irregular heartbeat). The attendant problems surrounding abnormal blood pressure, whether low or high, such as a ringing in the ears, some visual defects and dizziness caused by the blood rushing to the head after sudden movement, disappear with regular use of Mistletoe tea.

It is said that if a woman takes Mistletoe regularly, her monthly menses will be without cramping and any abnormally heavy menstruation will be regulated. In addition, after taking Mistletoe tea for some years, menopause will create no difficulties and hot flashes, anxieties which plague certain menopausal females, and heart palpitations will not occur. One old country legend which has not been verified states that 25 drops of the fresh juice of Mistletoe taken in water before breakfast and again after breakfast will render a barren women fertile.

As one final note of importance to women, I would like to remark on a recent study showing that a high percentage of women over 50 years of age who have been taking medication for high blood pressure for a period of time develop cancer of the breast. Mistletoe acts to normalize blood pressure and might therefore be considered to be an important adjunct to the medication.

Anyone suffering from a metabolic disorder, hormonal imbalance or any kind of upset of the glands is thought to benefit from Mistletoe's ability to normalize the body. Mistletoe is believed by many herbalists to possess remarkable properties which act favorably on the pancreas. For this reason alone, Mistletoe may be a valuable aid to diabetics. Two cups of the cold infusion daily are usually suggested for the above conditions, to be sipped morning and evening.

And at least one European herbalist believes in Mistletoe's legendary powers against epilepsy and suggests its use for nervous complaints of all kinds

TRADITIONAL USE - EXTERNALLY: Mistletoe possesses the ability to promote rapid clotting of the blood. Sniffing a cold infusion of the herb may stop a nosebleed and speed healing of the membranes.

As related in the text, Mistletoe ointment is of good use in the case of chilblains, even of long-standing origin.

HOW TO PREPARE MISTLETOE AS A COLD INFUSION: In proportions of 1 heaping teaspoon to every 6 ounces of cold water, soak Mistletoe leaves and twigs overnight. The following morning, warm gently and strain into a cup. You might find it efficient to keep the warmed tea in a thermos during the day if taking it in quantity.

HOW TO PREPARE MISTLETOE JUICE: Wash a quantity of fresh leaves and small twigs, taking care not to include any berries. While the herb parts are still wet, run through a juice extractor.

HOW TO PREPARE MISTLETOE OINTMENT: In order to retain as much liquid as possible, crush a quantity of fresh Mistletoe berries directly into a small amount of pure lard (not vegetable shortening) with a fork. Blend in well and store under refrigeration.

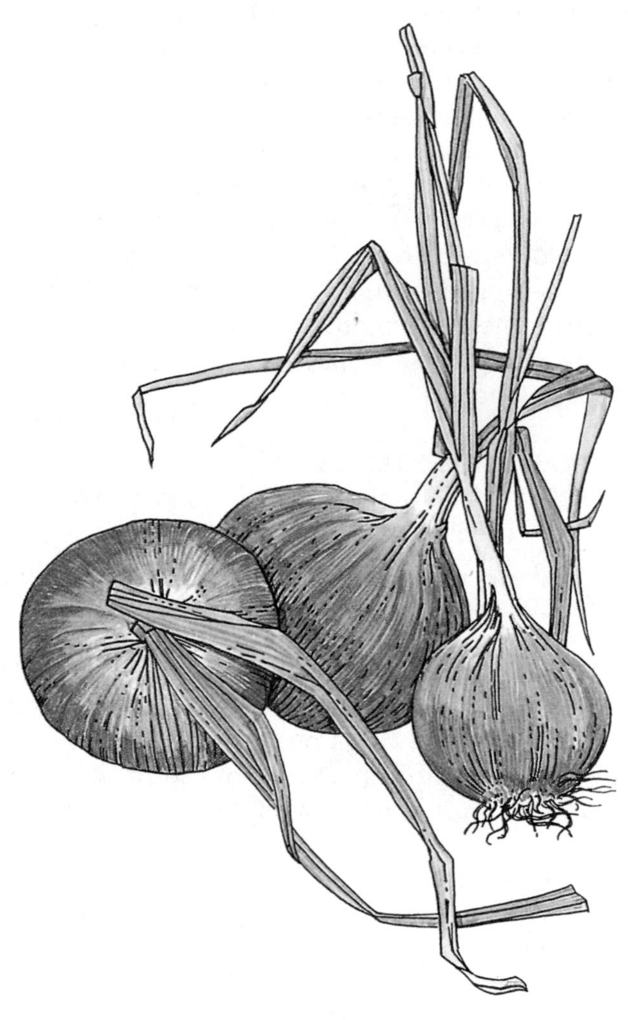

Onion

Allium cepa

Chapter 23
ONION
(Allium cepa)

Appetite (weak)
Asthma
Blood Clots
Blood-Sugar
Blood Pressure (high)
Blood (purifier)
Bronchitis
Catarrh (nasal)
Chilblains
Colds
Coughs
Coronary Thrombosis
Digestive Tract
Digestive Aid
Diuretic
Dizziness
Ears (ringing in)
Frostbite
Gas (flatulence)
Heart (strengthens)
Insect Bites
Longevity
Mouth (purifier
Phlebitis
Pneumonia (early)
Throat (sore)
Wounds (supperating)

PAST HISTORY: It is commonly believed the onion is a native of Egypt. Like its 'kissin' cousin,' garlic, the onion has been documented as a favorite food of the early pyramid-building Egyption slaves. The famed Greek historian, Herodotus, tells us that nine tons of gold were needed as payment for the incredible quantities of onions consumed by the hard-working slaves.

Egyptian pharoahs and priests revered both the onion and garlic bulbs. Surviving mosaics, hieroglyphs and paintings dating back to about 3200-2780 B.C. depict Egyptian royalty and priests in ceremonial acts involving the onion. The brown skin which covers the onion bulb was thought to be a symbol of the universe.

An early herbal says of the onion, "Boiled they give a kindly relish, raise appetites, corroborate the Stomach, cut Phlegm and profit the Asthmatical." Master Herbalist Culpepper agrees and notes, "The onion is so common and well known it needs no description. Onions increase sperm, especially the seed. They kill worms in children if they drink the water wherein they have been steeped all night. Being roasted under the embers and eaten with honey or sugar and oil, they much conduce to help an inveterate cough and expectorate tough phlegm. When plentifully eaten, they procure sleep, help digestion, cure acid belchings, remove obstructions and increase urinary secretions."

DESCRIPTION & GROWING REQUIREMENTS: As far as their medicinal qualities go, all onions are created equal. If you wish to grow your own, by far the most efficient method is to procure 'onion sets' in the spring and place them in your own garden. Any nursery can supply you with these tiny plants and they are singularly easy to grow as long as the soil is well worked and porous.

HOW TO HARVEST & STORE: Dig out the bulbs in the late fall, brush off the earth, and set aside to dry. It's fun to braid a few strings of bulbs and hang them in the kitchen where you may pluck off one or two as needed. It might amuse you to know in so doing you will be emulating many London householders of ages past who believed onions in the home could clear the evil humors from the air and keep them free of the dreaded Black Plague.

LEGENDARY USES: Do onions contain elements which retard the aging process? Many modern researchers believe both onions and garlic contribute to longevity. The following story tends to give credence to this theory.

A Turkish gentleman by the name of Zora Agha is said to have attained the ripe old age of 142 years by eating only one meal per day. This meal, which he ate daily with great pleasure, consisted mainly of coarse black bread and raw onions, which he crunched into and ate in-hand, rather as we eat an apple.

When Zora Agha was 140 years of age, his fame was so great that he was brought to the U.S. by an entrepreneur who exhibited him on an arduous tour around the country. According to a number of reports, this vigorous old gentlemen enjoyed the sights as much as Americans enjoyed seeing him. Unfortunately, the common diet of the U.S. proved too much for him. After partaking of meat for the first time in his life and eating his meals in a restaurant for two years during the tour, Zora Agha died.

TRADITIONAL USE - INTERNALLY: Regular use of the onion in whatever form you choose is said to purify the blood, invigorate the heart, lower high-blood pressure and normalize elevated blood-sugar. Onions stimulate gastric secretions, improve digestion, increase a flagging appetite and eliminate gas.

The documented bactericidal action of the onion aids in preventing putrefaction and fermentation in the digestive tract. Eating a raw onion has been shown to eliminate all bacteria in the mouth. As a good diuretic, the onion promotes the flow of urine, thereby reducing bloat and swelling of the extremities.

The onion is an almost legendary aid in conquering the common cold, helps dispel coughs, bronchitis, nasal catarrh, ear-ringing, dizziness and relieves asthma. One of the earliest forms of 'cough syrup,' still highly effective against coughs, colds and bronchitis, is a teaspoon of Onion Syrup every two or three hours. See instructions under 'How to Prepare' at the close of the chapter.

In the case of onions, medical science is beginning to pay attention to the herbalists. In fact, recent research abroad (Britain) has demonstrated that onions help increase the body's ability to prevent or dissolve internal clots which may cause phlebitis or break free and pass through the heart in a deadly form of coronary thrombosis. American scientists have identified and isolated *prostaglandin* in onions. This hormone is employed medically to lower high blood pressure. And French doctors have effectively used onions in a three-day treatment designed to eliminate fluid in the cardiac and pleural sacs.

TRADITIONAL USE - EXTERNALLY: Onion poultices have been used since time immemorial for sore throats, frostbite, chilblains, insect bites and as a healing against for supperating wounds. Traditional herbalists swear by raw onion slices glazed with cold-pressed olive oil as a specific to ward off beginning pneumonia and to treat an annoying dry cough.

HOW TO ENJOY THE ONION AS PREVENTIVE: Try Zora Agha's method of eating a raw onion daily (sliced, if you like) with a good whole- grain bread. Or simply have a bowl of hearty onion soup along with dark bread.

HOW TO PREPARE ONION "TEA:" Chop finely a medium onion and soak for 24-hours in 8 ounces of fresh cold water. Strain off the residue and drink the entire quantity over a period of 48 hours.

HOW TO PREPARE ONION SYRUP: Place thinly sliced onions in a heavy crock and layer alternately with a thick sprinkling of sugar.

Allow the mixture to remain undisturbed overnight. The following day, pour off the syrup and take as suggested in the text. This syrup will remain potent for three days.

HOW TO PREPARE THE ONION AS DIURETIC: Chop one medium onion and simmer in 8 ounces of water to which 2 tablespoons of honey have been added. After five minutes, remove from heat and strain off the residue. Take 3 or 4 tablespoons three times daily. If you pass dark or bloody urine, see a physician immediately for a urinalysis.

HOW TO PREPARE AN ONION POULTICE: Thickly slice a medium onion and heat over low heat in a little olive-oil. When warmed through, wrap in a light cloth or gauze and place on the affected area. Cover immediately with plastic-wrap (a bread-bag will work) to retain the heat and wrap warmly. Hint: To take away the hurt from a bee, wasp or insect sting, a slice of raw onion applied to the area draws out the pain almost immediately.

Chapter 24
PLANTAIN - RIBWORT
(Plantago lanceolata)

Asthma
Bedsores
Bite (human/dog)
Bladder
Blood (purifier)
Bronchitis
Cancer (skin)
Cancer (glandular)
Coughs
Detoxifier
Digestive Tract
Extremities (swollen)
Hoarseness
Infection
Insect Bites
Kidneys
Limb (amputated)
Liver
Lungs (weak)
Respiratory Disorders
Skin Irritations
Snakebite
Sores (open)
Wounds (puncture)

PAST HISTORY: The Plantain family of Plantaginaceae contains more than 200 species and at least twenty-five or thirty of these have been used medicinally for centuries. The most important of the species are Plantago lanceolata and Plantago major, the common and the Broad-Leaved Plantain respectively.

In one of the oldest sources of early Anglo-Saxon medicine, the *Lacnunga*, Weybroed (Plantain) is listed as one of the nine sacred herbs and is the prime ingredient of a 'salve for flying venom,' undoubtedly a reference to the belief that the leaves of the Plantain are a remedy against the bite of a rattlesnake or mad dog. One of the old Herbals says, "If a wood hound (mad dog) rend a man, take this wort, rub it fine and lay it on and then will the spot soon be whole."

Gower, a physician of the 12th century, calls Plantain "the herb sovereine," and Salmon's Herbal of 1710 lists many uses for Plantain in these words: "The liquid juice clarified and drunk for several days helps distillation of rheum upon the throat, glands, lungs. An especial remedy against ulceration of the lungs and a vehement cough arising from same. It is said to be good against epilepsy, dropsy, jaundice and opens obstructions of the liver, spleen and veins. Dropt into the ears, it eases their pains and restores hearing much decayed."

Plantain is in still wide use around the world by herbalists who praise its powers. In the Scottish Highlands yet today, Plantain is called *Slan-lus*, plant of healing.

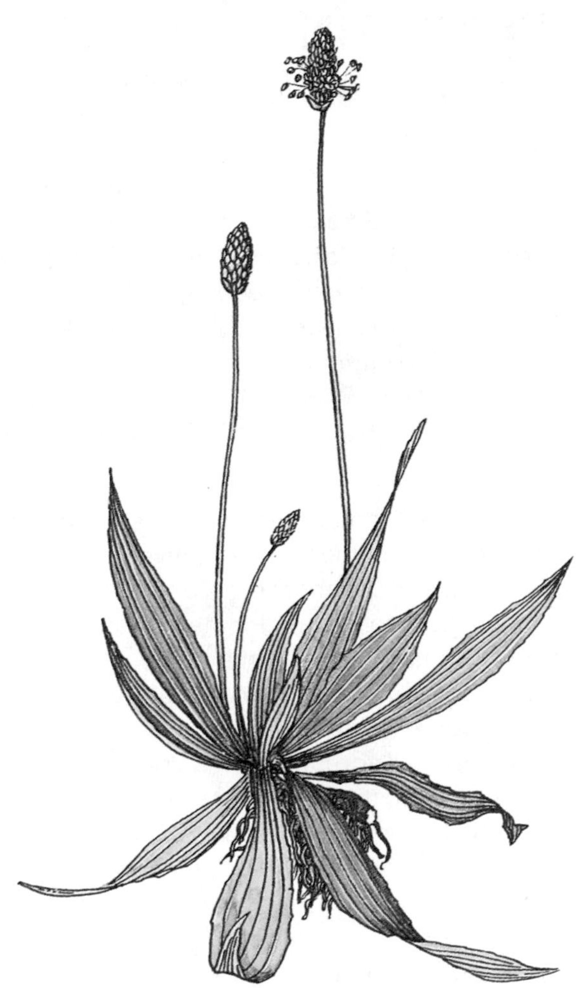

Plantain — Ribwort

Plantago lanceolata

DESCRIPTION & GROWING REQUIREMENTS: Often called 'Snakeweed,' the Ribwort Plantain is a tall slender plant with rather narrow dark-green leaf blades which often attain a length of more than a foot. When the ribbed blades sway in the breeze, they do indeed resemble a snake about to strike, but the common name of 'Snakeweed' refers instead to Plantain's legendary curative powers rather than its appearance. The flower-stalks are even taller and terminate in dense spikes.

The Broad-Leaved Plantain bears an equally tall flower stalk, but its leaves form a rosette around the base of the herb and can be anywhere from four to 10 inches long, with the leaves being about two-thirds as broad as they are long. The early term for Plantain, 'Weybroed' (or Way-Bread) refers to the fact that the Plantains were found flourishing along the 'King's Way,' as the highways of the time were known.

This hasn't changed. Plantains may still be found growing happily along roads and in country pastures. If you bring some home, be aware that this plant is easily transplanted but not as easily controlled. The Plantains have a way of encroaching on neighboring plantings.

HOW TO HARVEST & STORE: Although the entire herb - leaves, flowers, seeds and roots - has medicinal qualities, the fresh leaves are most often used in various preparations. In order to have Plantain available year-around, you may wish to prepare a strong infusion (see directions for preparation at the close of the chapter) and freeze in ice-cube trays for later use. Once the tea is solidly frozen, empty the cubes into a freezer bag and close tightly. You will also find directions for preparing two Plantain honeys at the close of the chapter.

LEGENDARY CURES: It seems farmers and all country folk know of the infection-fighting and healing properties of Plantain. I was talking across the fence one day not long ago with a neighbor, Robert K., who was raking up debris and clearing a space for a kitchen garden when he slipped and came down hard on the tines of his rake with one hand, leaving two deep puncture wounds in the fleshy part of his palm.

Although I'm a strong believer in the healing powers of Nature's Pharmacy, I offered to drive him in to get a tetanus shot, knowing the dangers of puncture wounds. He laughed and pulled off a fresh Plantain leaf. He then balled it up in his uninjured hand and squeezed juice directly into the two small holes in his injured hand, which he first pinched to drive blood to the surface. Even though the leaf was unwashed and dirty from the field, his hand healed cleanly and no infection developed.

Robert K. also told me of his brother's son who had an arm amputated because of a war injury. The stump pained him constantly and developed open sores which refused to heal. Because of these raw sores, he couldn't wear his artificial arm and consequently wasn't able to hold down a job for long. The family lived in a different state, but at a family reunion one year, Robert went out into the fields and came back with some Plantain leaves which he crushed and applied to the young man's painful stump. Robert told me his nephew termed it a miracle when the raw, open sores began to close and heal almost overnight. The young man is now able to wear his prosthesis and has a good paying job.

From a particularly reliable source come two other stories of Plantain's miraculous powers. One concerns an elderly woman, Jocelyn Y., who had suffered for close to twenty years with open sores on her feet. Because of the danger of infection, this woman never went out of the house. Even these very old sores yielded to Plantain within a few weeks. It appears the healing was permanent. According to my source, even after six months, the wounds had not reopened.

The other story concerns a woman who developed a hard lump on her upper arm after having been bitten by a child. Her name escapes me now, but she dabbed fresh Plantain juice on the lump and it softened and eventually disappeared.

TRADITIONAL USE - INTERNALLY: Both the old Herbals and modern herbalists agree that the Plantains are particularly useful for all respiratory disorders, including weak lungs, hoarseness, chronic coughs, bronchitis and even bronchial asthma.

For these conditions and for kidney involvement, the accepted method of ingestion is to bring to a boil 6 ounces of cold water with a slice of lemon and a heaping teaspoon of raw honey. When just boiling, remove from the fire and stir in 1 teapoon of freshly minced Plantain leaves. Steep, covered, for 30 seconds and sip as hot as possible. This tea may be taken up to five cups daily if the condition is serious.

If bronchial asthma or liver or bladder infections are the problem, the addition of 1 heaping teaspoon Thyme (see Chapter 31) to the above mixture is recommended.

The Plantains are also said to aid in cleansing the blood, the lungs and the entire digestive tract. To rid the body of toxins, it is usually suggested that adults take 1 tablespoonful of Plantain honey (1 teaspoon for children) directly before each of the three daily meals for three weeks.

It is interesting to note that ancient physicians believed Plantain seeds to be the finest of all preventive measures against the development of kidney or bladder stones.

TRADITIONAL USE - EXTERNALLY: Crushed or bruised Plantain leaves appear to contain an infection-fighting element which makes them useful against open sores and wounds. All kinds of cuts, scratches, scrapes and stings are relieved by the application of these leaves. Human bites, dog bites and snake bites are treated by the traditionalists with Plantain leaves as well. Note: Any bite requires the immediate attention of a physician.

We have reports of European herbalists treating malignant growths (skin cancer) and malignant glandular disorders with Plantain leaves and Marjoram (see Chapter 20) oil. The oil is prepared by steeping fresh (or dried) Marjoram in olive oil for 10 days. This oil is then smoothed on the affected part of the body and the area is covered with crushed Plantain leaves and then lightly bandaged. Unfortunately, we have not been able to substantiate an actual cancer cure accomplished by this method.

The elderly who often suffer from bedsores or raw open sores which refuse to heal may be helped by a poultice of crushed Plantain leaves. The healing may be speeded by gently coating the edges of the wound with Calendula ointment (see Chapter 5) before applying the poultice. If there is swelling of the extremities, try a good soak of the affected limb in either Mallow (see Chapter 19) or Horsetail (see Chapter 18) before using the ointment and the poultice. This combination treatment has given very good results abroad.

HOW TO PREPARE PLANTAIN TEAS: Complete directions are given in the text above along with a description of the conditions which are relieved by the various mixtures.

HOW TO PREPARE A PLANTAIN POULTICE: Gather a quantity of fresh Plantain leaves. Wash well under cold running water and crush with a rolling pin directly onto a very clean white cloth in order not to lose the valuable juices. Apply as suggested above.

HOW TO PREPARE PLANTAIN HONEY: Heat to melt 2 cups of sugar, 1 cup of water and 2 cups of honey. Mince a quantity of freshly washed Plantain leaves and add a double handful to the sugar/honey blend. Simmer on low heat, stirring constantly, until the mixture thickens to a honey-like consistency. Pour into a clean glass jar, cover and store refrigerated.

HOW TO PREPARE PLANTAIN HONEY-WINE: In a heavy wide-mouthed crock, layer bruised Plantain leaves with raw sugar until the crock is almost full, pressing down well. After the layers settle, continue with alternate layers until the crock will hold no more. Cover the layers with several thicknesses of waxed paper and place a heavy weight on top. Put the crock in a warm place and allow it to remain undisturbed for three months. By this time, the jar will contain a quantity of fermented syrupy liquid. Put this juice through a fruit press and bring the resulting mixture to a full boil. Remove from heat, allow to cool and bottle.

Chapter 25
RADISH - BLACK
(Raphanus sativus)

Bile (promotes)
Bronchitis
Catarrh (intestinal)
Colds
Coughs
Diarrhea
Expectorant
Gall-Bladder
Gallstones
Gastrointestinal Aid
Hepatitis
Herpes Simplex
Insomnia
Liver
Mucous Membranes
Rheumatism
Sinuses
Scabies
Skin Conditions
Tonic

PAST HISTORY: All of the vegetables currently under cultivation by man stem from eight different regions of the world. The circuitous route taken by the radish to arrive at your table is shrouded in mystery, but the areas of the globe where the radish originated include central and western China, northwest India, Afghanistan and the U.S.S.R.

The radish has been cultivated since ancient times. Over 5,000 years ago, archaeological evidence shows that early Egyptians grew radishes along with crops of asparagus, cabbage, chard, celery, cucumbers, lettuce, peas and even watermelon.

Early herbals appear at times to confuse the radish (Raphanus sativus) with the root we now know as 'Horseradish' (Cochlearia Armoracia). The wild radish (Raphanos agrios) mentioned in early Greek writings has been variously identified as the black radish or the horseradish, depending on the source consulted. The London Pharmacopeia of the 18th century, *Materia Medica,*includes mention of Raphanus rusticanus but authorities generally agree the text refers to Horseradish.

DESCRIPTION & GROWING REQUIREMENTS: Forget about the little acorn-shaped red radishes you customarily slice into your salad. The black radish is its great-grandaddy! This root is hot and pungent, crisp white inside, with a thin blackish skin. It carries rough, stalked radial leaves and the blossoms may be white or pale violet. Like all root vegetables, the black radish likes well-worked ground. You will be rewarded with a fine table vegetable and healthy herb if you choose to

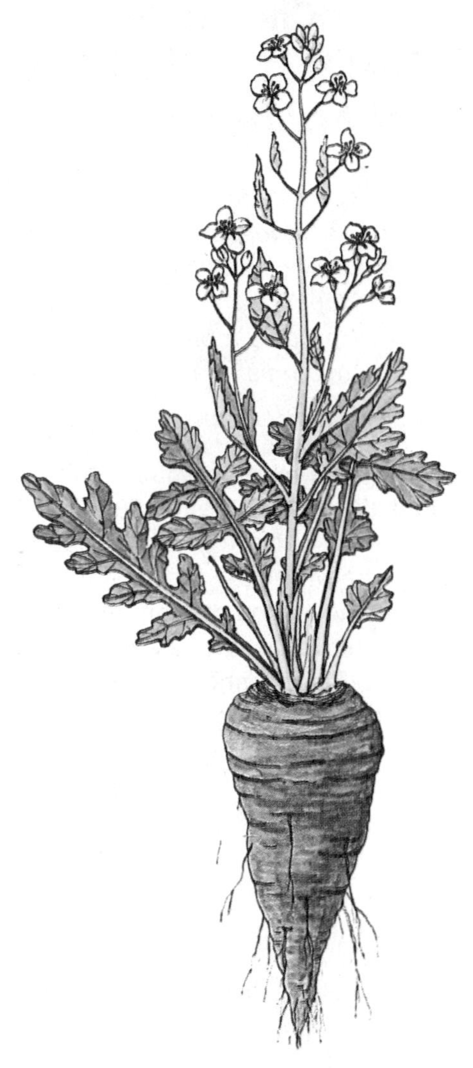

Radish — Black

Raphanus sativus

cultivate the black radish. We recommend it heartily both for its medicinal properties and delicious taste.

HOW TO HARVEST & STORE: The black radish comes to maturity early and may be harvested from May through October. If you wish, you may 'store' your crop in the ground where it grows by cutting down the tops and covering it over to protect it from frost. The roots will remain crisp and juicy for many months. Or, dig them out and place them in a box of sand in a dark, dry place.

LEGENDARY USE: I must confess that I remember the black radish 'spring cure' with great affection. This preventive is traditional in Europe and my grandmother raised a fine crop of black radishes on her Bavarian farm. It interests me to find the constituents of the black radish have now been identified by science as providing a form of health protection. The black radish 'spring cure' my great-grandmother handed down to grandmother is detailed at the close of the chapter under 'How to Prepare,' as closely as I can remember it.

TRADITIONAL USE - INTERNALLY: Fully one-third of the radish is natural potassium and it contains a high content of iron and magnesium as well. Both iron and magnesium are needed by the mucous membranes of the body. Folk medicine teaches that the entire radish family is rich in vitamins and minerals, but the black radish is clearly the most effective. With its content of sulpher-containing ethereal oil, the black radish is an excellent gastrointestinal stimulant, cleans the bile-ducts and encourages bile-flow at the same time. The black radish is traditionally used in Europe for all liver and gall-bladder complaints and is especially recommended for hepatitis and gall-stones.

The juice of the black radish makes a good expectorant and helps in bronchitis, coughs and colds and aids in clearing the sinuses of an accumulation of mucus. It has been successfully administered against intestinal catarrh, diarrhea and rheumatism. When the juice is taken over a long period of time, it is said to eliminate the itching of various skin conditions, such as herpes simplex and scabies. An an aid to the insomniac, an old folk saying goes: "Eat half a black radish a'fore going a'bed and sleep a'fore the pillow hits the head."

Note: When the black radish is used in conjunction with carrot juice, the combination of elements helps restore the tone of the mucous membranes of the entire body. Do not take the black radish alone if your stomach or intestines are inflamed. High intake may damage the mucosae of the gastrointestinal tract.

TRADITIONAL USE - EXTERNALLY: The black radish is a skin irritant and vesicant. It is not used externally.

TWO WAYS TO PREPARE THE BLACK RADISH 'SPRING CURE': (1) Thinly slice a quantity of the black radish root. Layer in a crock with a thick sprinkling of sugar. Allow the crock to stand undisturbed overnight. (2) Grate a quantity of black radish root and press to extract the juices. Add honey to taste.

Grandmother's Spring Cure: Take 1 to 2 tablespoons of the juice after the three meals of the day for seven days.

THE BLACK RADISH 'CURE': Using either method of preparation given above, take 2 tablespoons of the juice three times daily. Gradually increase your intake to a total of 1/2 cup juice taken three times daily until whatever ails you has been eliminated. Finish off the 'cure' by reducing your daily intake back to the original quantity of 2 tablespoons juice thrice daily.

THE BLACK RADISH 'PREVENTIVE': European country-folk enjoy unprecedented good health. A favorite meal is grated black radish heaped on a well-buttered slice of coarse, dark whole-grain bread.

Chapter 26
SAGE
(Salvia officinalis)

Abdominal Cramps
Appetite (weak)
Canker Sores
Coughs
Diarrhea
Digestive Tract
Gas (flatulence)
Glandular Disorders
Gingevitis
Gums (inflamed)
Expectorant
Insect Bites
Intestines (inflamed)
Limbs (paralyzed)
Liver
Mouth (ulcer)
Muscle Cramps
Nervous Complaints
Phlegm (tough)
Spinal Cord
Stress
Stroke
Sweats (night)
Teeth (loose)
Throat (sore)
Tonsillitis
*Tremors**

**All Age-Related Complaints*

PAST HISTORY: The common garden Sage, familiar as a flavoring in poultry stuffings, has been revered for its healing qualities since the earliest times. Its botanical name, Salvia, comes from the Latin *salvere,* meaning 'to be saved,' which was shortened variously to Sauja, then Sauge (French) and finally, in Old English, Sawge, leading to Sage, as we know it today.

An early Christian legend relates it was Sage who gave the Virgin Mary and the Baby Jesus shelter as they fled from Herod. When all danger was past, Mary told the Sage, "I give you power to heal mankind of all ills and save him from death as you have done for me."

Sage enjoyed such a strong reputation for its beneficial qualities that learned physicians of the Middle Ages were fond of saying, *"Cur moriatur homo cui Salvia crescit in horto?"* meaning *"Why should a man die whilst Sage grows in his garden?"* And a very old English proverb says, *"He that would live for aye, Must eat Sage in May."* This universal herb was praised in an old French saying, also: *"Sage helps the nerves and by its powerful might, Palsy is cured and fever put to flight."*

In fact, all the old Herbals extol the virtues of Sage. The famed Culpepper himself had this to say, "Good for diseases of the liver and to make blood. Sage provokes urine and stayeth the bleeding of wounds and cleaneth ulcers and sores. The juice of Sage with vinegar

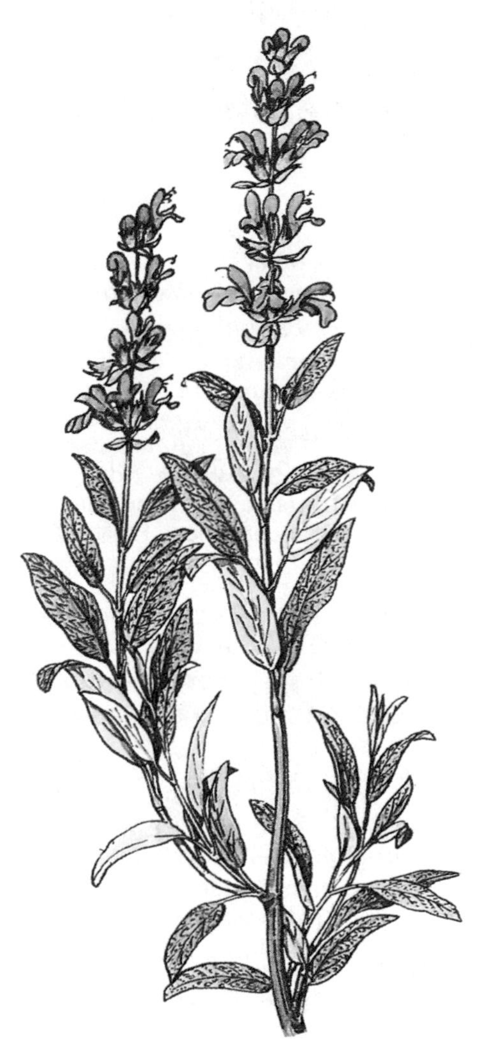

Sage

Salvia officinalis

and honey put thereto is used to wash sore mouths and throats, as need requireth." Modern herbalists agree.

DESCRIPTION & GROWING REQUIREMENTS: Sage blossoms in late summer and puts forth grayish-purple flowers with a strong pleasant scent. The herb grows about a foot high with the silvery-green leaves set in pairs on wiry stems.

Sage prefers a sheltered partially sunny location and, in some climates, may need to be covered against the cold of winter. Sage is exceptionally easy to cultivate and deserves a place of honor in your herb garden.

HOW TO HARVEST & STORE: Gather the leaves before the blossoms mature by pinching them off. Be sure to bring in the harvest while the sun is high and bright. The volatile oils of this herb are at their most potent at midday. Dry the leaves on a screen in a warm, airy place. When the flowers are fully open, gather them also for the making of Sage vinegar. (See 'How to Prepare' at the close of this chapter.)

LEGENDARY CURES: The writings of a modern British herbalist tell of a Mrs. Jane D. who related how Sage acted on a severe bout of tonsillitis afflicting her son, Tom. When Tom awakened one morning with inflamed and obviously infected tonsils, Mrs. D. prepared a tea of Sage and had Tom use the infusion as a deep gargle every other hour all day long.

By the following morning, Tom's tonsils were back to normal. Mrs. D. said Tom was prone to tonsilitis and often missed school because of it. She was flabbergasted at his speedy recovery with the Sage gargle and has resolved never to be without Sage in her household again.

The Chinese, expert herbalists for thousands of years, regard Sage as the remedy of choice to ward off the stresses of old age. A good example of this use concerns the story of a hard-working man, Keith W. Although Mr. W. was only in his mid-fifties his doctor had recommended he take an early retirement, saying he wouldn't be responsible if Mr. W. insisted on keeping up his usual pace. His nerves were raw and he raged at his family constantly because the stress of running a successful business single-handedly for many years had taken its toll.

As a stop-gap measure, Mr. W. finally agreed to take a vacation, but insisted all he needed was a little rest. While on vacation at Martha's Vineyard, he met a singularly spry and energetic woman of some seventy-five years of age. She confided to him that she took a cup of Sage tea after meals every day and believed that was what kept her so young and active. The kindly old lady gave Mr. W. some fresh Sage leaves and he promptly began the treatment himself. His condition was long-standing and deteriorating, but I am pleased to report that after six months on Sage tea, Mr. W. received a clean bill of health from his doctor.

TRADITIONAL USE - INTERNALLY: Traditional herbalists and some European physicians believe Sage is helpful in cases of cramps, the tremors of the aged, glandular problems and even minor disorders of the spinal cord. Taken frequently, Sage strengthens the system, may help prevent the onset of a stroke and is beneficial to the paralytic. For these disorders, at least two cups of Sage tea are suggested daily.

With its cleansing properties, Sage can be valuable in liver complaints and is said to benefit the entire digestive tract by eliminating gas, conquering diarrhea and soothing inflamed intestines. Sage is an excellent expectorant and aids coughing up unhealthy phlegm. The convalescent recovers his appetite on Sage tea and this tea eliminates 'night sweats' as well.

Medical science is no longer removing tonsils 'wholesale' as they used to do in the past, now recognizing the tonsils as the local and relatively easily treated repository of the body for most toxins. Unfortunately, those of us who had a tonsillectomy in our youth find these toxins now settle in the kidneys. Remember to take Sage tea in all cases of throat and tonsil infections.

TRADITIONAL USE — EXTERNALLY: In addition to the internal treatment, an infusion of Sage is of immense benefit as a gargle or mouthwash for sore throat or infected tonsils. A canker sore and ulcers of the mouth and throat are soothed and healed by swishing Sage tea around the affected parts. Loose teeth, bleeding gums, gingevitis (infected and receeding gums) and inflamed gums yield to a regular thrice daily use of Sage tea as a mouthwash.

Women who suffer abdominal cramps and anyone with a nervous

complaint will find relief by taking a Sage sitz bath. As a final note, crushed fresh Sage leaves take the sting out of insect and bug bites of all types.

HOW TO PREPARE A SAGE INFUSION: Pour 6 ounces of freshly boiled water over 1 level teaspoon of the herb (fresh or dried leaves) and steep, covered, for a few minutes. Strain, sweeten with honey, if you like, and sip hot.

HOW TO PREPARE SAGE VINEGAR: Fill a glass bottle with freshly picked Sage flowers and add enough apple-cider vinegar to completely cover the blossoms. Cork the bottle loosely and allow it to remain in a warm place for two weeks. A teaspoon of this blend taken after meals is a well-known aid to healthy digestion.

HOW TO PREPARE A SAGE SITZ BATH: Steep two heaping double handfuls of fresh or dried leaves in 2 quarts of cold water overnight. The following day, boil the mixture, strain off the residue and add the liquid to your bath.

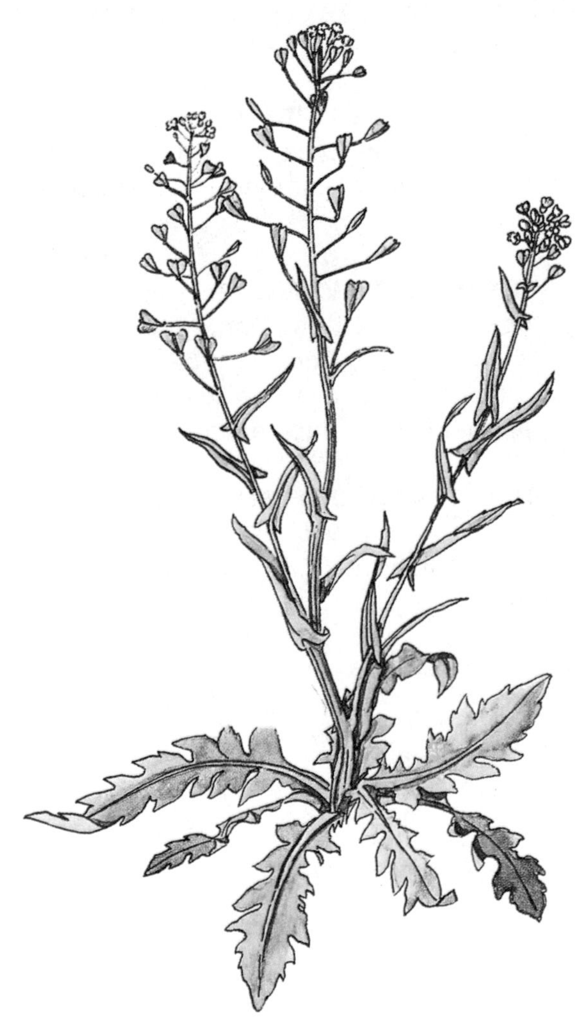

Shepherd's Purse

Capsella bursa-pastoris

Chapter 27
SHEPHERD'S PURSE
(Capsella bursa-pastoris)

Bleeding (internal)
Bleeding (external)
Blood Pressure
Breasts (swollen)
Hemorrhoids
Hernia
Hot-Flashes
Menstruation (heavy)
Menstruation (irregular)
Menopause
Muscular Atrophy
Muscular Disorders
Nervous Complaints
Rectum (prolapsed)
Wounds

PAST HISTORY: Shepherd's Purse is considered the most important medicinal from the family Cruciferae. Shepherd's Purse was so named because its flat little seed-pouches do indeed resemble an old-fashioned snap-top change purse. In France, it is known as *Bourse de pasteur* and in Ireland, Shepherd's Purse is called *Clappedepouch* after the lepers who were required to announce their condition with a clapper. The lepers, who begged for their sustenance, received their alms in a cup fastened to the end of a long pole lest they infect those on whose charity they were dependent.

The master herbalist, Culpepper, says Shepherd's Purse "Helps bleeding from wounds, inward or outward, and if made into poultices, helps inflammation and St. Anthony's fire (a severe inflammation or gangrenous skin condition). The juice dropt into the ears heals the pains, noise and matterings thereof. If it be bound to the wrists or soles of the feet, it helps the jaundice."

The hemostyptic (blood-clotting) qualities of Shepherd's Purse have long been recognized. In World War I, a liquid extract of *Capsella bursa-pastoris* was in much demand by the doctors and was used to stop both internal and external bleeding of all kinds.

DESCRIPTION & GROWING REQUIREMENTS: This persistent herb grows everywhere and, like the Dandelion, is often regarded as a weed by those unversed in herbal lore who consider it fit only to be uprooted and eradicated. The leaves of the Shepherd's Purse are irregularly toothed and resemble those of the Dandelion, forming a rosette around the lower part of the branched stem.

You will often see a Shepherd's Purse bearing tiny off-white flowers on the top half of the stem with seed pouches on the lower half. The flowers go to seed in the order of their appearance, with the very last flower still in blossom at the tip of the long slender stem and the balance covered with little leathery 'purses.'

Shepherd's Purse is not particular as to its location and can flourish almost anywhere. When all conditions are right and it is rooted in rich top soil, it may grow as tall as three feet. Where it clings to life in poor, rocky soil, it may be only inches high.

HOW TO HARVEST & STORE: Because Shepherd's Purse is most powerful fresh, this is a very valuable planting in the home herb garden. The entire herb, leaves, stems, flowers and seed 'purses' are used. You may prepare a strong infusion (see 'How to Prepare' at the close of the chapter) and freeze cubes for storage. Once the tea is solidly frozen, place the cubes in a freezer bag and close tightly. It is a simple matter to thaw a cube quickly in hot water for fresh tea when needed. You will also find directions for preparing a Tincture of Shepherd's Purse at the close of the chapter. The tincture stores very well.

LEGENDARY CURES: A particularly interesting and somewhat mystical story coming from Germany relates of a renowned German herbalist who was gifted with an old hand-written diary of herbal remedies. Because the herbalist followed a very heavy schedule, the old herbal was put to one side and almost forgotten. The herbalist awakened suddenly one dark midnight from a sound sleep and felt impelled to look through the old book. Settling down comfortably, the herbalist opened the yellowing pages and found a hitherto unknown method of help for muscular atrophy. Marking the single passage well, the herbalist returned to bed and immediately fell back into a dreamless sleep.

A few days later, a phone call came with a plea for help from a registered nurse who had been forced to stop work because she suffered a peculiar form of muscular atrophy. The herbalist immediately recalled the old herb remedy and told the nurse how to prepare Shepherd's Purse tincture, instructing her to massage it briskly into the affected limbs. The patient was also told to drink four cups of Lady's Mantle tea (see Chapter 19) daily.

A month later, the herbalist and the nurse compared notes. On the very night the herbalist was impelled to leaf through the old herbal where the specific treatment needed was found, the nurse had made a religious pilgrimage seeking help for her condition. After her prayers, a man came up to her in the street and told her to contact the herbalist, which she did with such spectacular results. The nurse was so strengthened and healed that she is once again a practicing nurse after two years of suffering. It may be well and truly said that God works in mysterious ways!

Another combination of herbs worked wonders for an elderly woman who had a weak anus muscle which caused a prolapse of the rectum. The woman suffered agonizing pain in the entire abdominal area. Despite two surgical operations, the condition was not corrected. Four cups of Lady's Mantle tea taken daily to strengthen the internal muscles was recommended, along with a brisk massage with Shepherd's Purse tincture of the affected area. Because ten days are required to bring the tincture to maturity, a Swedish Bitters (see Chapter 30) compress was suggested for the interim. Just a few days after beginning the treatment, the woman reported her pain was fading. Within a month, her anus muscle began functioning normally and eventually even the prolapsed rectum was healed.

Even more astounding was the reported cure of a hernia without surgical intervention. A busy farmwife used compresses of Swedish Bitters, massaged with Shepherd's Purse tincture and drank four cups of Lady's Mantle tea daily while wearing a support. After two months, all pain was gone along with all signs of the hernia, much to the surprise of her doctor who had urged an operation.

TRADITIONAL USE — INTERNALLY: As was noted earlier, Shepherd's Purse has even been recognized medically as of superior benefit in staunching bleeding of all kinds. Whether from wounds suffered in battle, or from nose, stomach, intestinal or uterine bleeding, two to three cups of Shepherd's Purse tea taken daily is immensely effective. For bleeding from the kidneys, the addition of an equal amount of Horsetail (see Chapter 18) to the Shepherd's Purse is recommended when preparing the infusion.

To normalize an excessive menstrual flow, two cupfuls of Shepherd's Purse tea daily taken during the ten days before the expected onset of menstruation is recommended. An irrregular menstrual flow of a young woman entering puberty may be regulated in the same manner. After menopause, to eliminate the discomfort of menopausal problems, a woman will benefit by taking two cupfuls daily for a period of four weeks. Stop the treatment for the following three weeks and begin again for another four weeks. It is said this course of treatment will soothe the nerves and eliminate hot flashes.

Shepherd's Purse, like Mistletoe (see Chapter 21), regulates blood pressure, stabilizing and normalizing the pressure, whether low or high. Two cups daily are suggested, to be taken only until the pressure is normalized.

TRADITIONAL USE — EXTERNALLY: A cold decoction of Shepherd's Purse applied to an open wound will prove most effective. Refer to the text above for use of Shepherd's Purse tincture as a friction rub and massage aid for all muscular disorders and atrophy. For burning and bleeding hemorrhoids, a small enema with a warm infusion of Shepherd's Purse brings blessed relief. A sitz bath is also of benefit for this condition and offers immediate help.

A nursing mother suffering from painful and swollen breasts will be eased with a compress of fresh Shepherd's Purse applied warm. This is a very comforting treatment.

HOW TO PREPARE A SHEPHERD'S PURSE INFUSION: Pour 6 ounces of freshly boiled water over 1 heaping teaspoon of the herb. Cover and steep for a few minutes. Strain and sweeten with honey if desired.

HOW TO PREPARE A SHEPHERD'S PURSE TINCTURE: Gather a quantity of the fresh whole herb. Finely mince the flowers, leaves, stems and seed pods and place loosely in a clean glass bottle. Pour in spirits to cover and put the bottle in a warm place for ten days. Use as suggested in the text.

HOW TO PREPARE A SHEPHERD'S PURSE COMPRESS: Gather a quantity of the fresh whole herb. Finely mince the flowers, leaves, stems and seed pods and place in a large strainer over rapidly boiling water. Cover and allow the hot steam to wilt and penetrate every healing morsel. Turn the warm, moist herb onto a clean white cloth and fold the cloth around it. Apply to the affected area.

HOW TO PREPARE A SHEPHERD'S PURSE SITZ BATH: Gather a quantity of the fresh whole herb. Chop coarsely and steep a heaping double handful in two quarts of fresh cold water over night. The following morning, bring to a boil and strain off the residue. Add to a sitz (or full) bath.

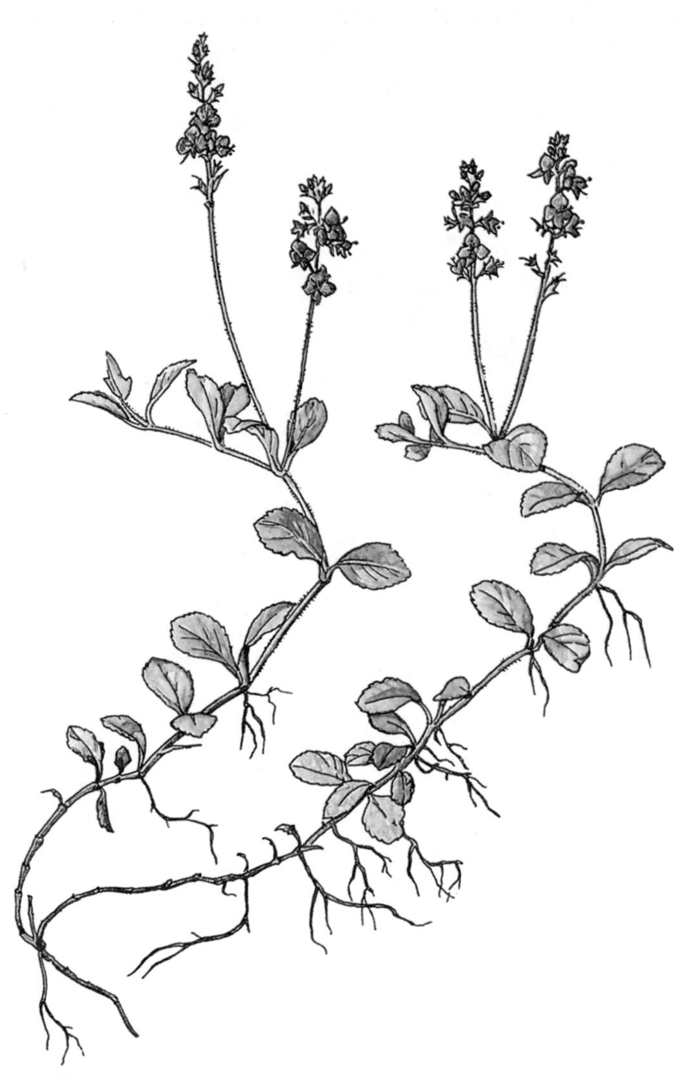

Speedwell

Veronica officinalis

Chapter 28
SPEEDWELL
(Veronica officinalis)

Blood (purifier)
Bronchitis
Bursitis
Cholesterol
Concentration Aid
Cough
Digestive Tract
Dizziness
Eczema
Gout
Intestinal Problems
Jaundice
Liver Complaints
Memory Lapses
Mental Over-Exertion
Nervous Complaints
Phlegm (tough)
Pruritis (senile)
Rheumatism
Skin Conditions
Spleen Disorders
Stress
Wounds (infected)
Wounds (inflamed)

PAST HISTORY: The name 'Speedwell' may seem to speak for itself, but at least one old herbal states the name comes from the fragility of the herb which drops its leaves at the slightest touch. Country folk of days of old often called the herb 'Farewell' or 'Goodbye' because the leaves said'farewell' to the stem so quickly.

Although many modern herbals omit any mention of Speedwell, this species of Veronica had a respected place among recognized remedies until the comparatively recent past. All the ancient herbals give Speedwell a place of honor and speak highly of its value as a purifier of the blood and a remedy of note in various skin disorders. In days of old, Speedwell was believed to be a cure for both the dreaded smallpox and measles. Gerard, certainly one of the most celebrated of the early herbalists, recommended Speedwell for cancer, "to be given in the broth of a hen" (our modern-day cure-all, chicken soup), and advocated the root as a specific against pestilential fevers.

Roman physicians valued the virtues of Speedwell to such a great degree and used it so effectively that a common compliment of the times was to say an individual had as many virtues as the Speedwell.

DESCRIPTION & GROWING REQUIREMENTS: Speedwell is a perennial which bears clusters of pale blue flowers that rise up from creeping hairy stems that can be anywhere from three to eighteen inches long, depending on whether or not its environment is favorable. Its tiny toothed leaves appear silvery green and run in pairs the length of the stem. Speedwell can be found growing wild along the edges of woodland paths and in pastures.

Select a rather dry, partially sunny location in your garden for Speedwell where it has room for its wandering ways. If you have an oak tree, so much the better. This herb seems to draw strength from the oak and Speedwells found growing near the mighty oak have the mightiest powers.

HOW TO HARVEST & STORE: This is another herb whose powers are greatly diminished in the dried form. Fortunately, Speedwell has a long growing season and flowers from early spring to late summer. The entire plant is medicinal, but must be harvested when in flower. If the leaves fall from the stem, gather them from the ground and bring them home also.

Speedwell stimulates the entire digestive tract and is gentle in action, making it suitable for the young and aged alike. Intestinal complaints often yield to Speedwell and it assists in the bringing up or passing of mucus and phlegm. One teaspoon of the fresh juice taken after each of the three daily meals helps the healing of eczema and is especially suggested for senile pruritis. A tincture of Speedwell, 15 drops in water thrice daily, often eases the pain of rheumatism, bursitis and gout.

TRADITIONAL USE — EXTERNALLY: In addition to taking the tincture internally, a brisk massage of the affected areas with the tincture greatly assists in relieving the pain of rheumatism, bursitis and gout.

Inflamed and infected wounds which refuse to heal benefit by a gentle cleansing with an infusion of Speedwell. Finish the treatment by using the infusion as a well-warmed well-wrapped overnight compress.

HOW TO PREPARE SPEEDWELL TINCTURE: Gather a quantity of the fresh herb, flowers, leaves and stems. Mince finely (scissors make it easy) and put two heaping handfuls of the herb in a quart glass (not plastic) bottle. Fill to cover with spirits and allow to remain undisturbed in a warm place for two weeks.

HOW TO PREPARE FRESH JUICE: Gather a quantity of the fresh flower heads and leaves. Wash very gently under cold running water and place in the juice extractor still dripping. You may bottle the juice and store in the refrigerator.

HOW TO PREPARE SPEEDWELL INFUSION (TEA): Use 1 heaping teaspoon for each 6 ounces of freshly boiled water. Steep, covered, for three or four minutes. Strain, sweeten with a little honey and sip hot.

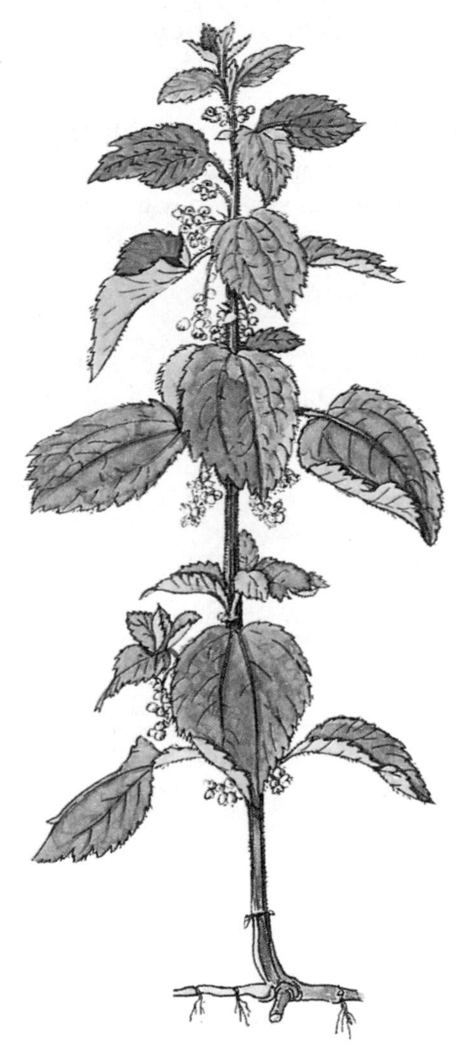

Stinging Nettle
Urtica dioica

Chapter 29
STINGING NETTLE
(Urtica dioica)

Allergies
Anemia
Arthritis
Asthma
Bactericide
Blood (builder)
Blood Disorders
Blood (purifier)
Blood Sugar
Bursitis
Cancer (abdominal)
Chlorosis
Circulatory Problems
Colds
Dandruff
Diabetes
Diuretic
Eczema
Fatigue (chronic)
Fungicide
Gall Bladder
Hair (thinning)
Hay Fever
Headaches (severe)
Hyperglycemia
Hypoglycemia
Infections
Leukemia
Liver
Pancreas
Respiratory Tract
Rheumatism
Sciatica
Skin Conditions
Stomach Cramps
Tonic
Ulcers (internal)
Ulcer (skin)
Urinary Tract
Vascular Aid
Viricide

PAST HISTORY: The Stinging Nettle family contains about 500 species and has a singularly interesting history. According to old writings, the Stinging Nettle was introduced to Britain by the conquering Romans. Camden, in his historical work *Britannica,* says, "The soldiers brought some of the nettle seed with them and sowed it there for their use to rub and chafe their limbs, when through extreme cold they should be benumbed, having been told the climate of Britain was so cold it could not be endured."

The common name is said to come from the Anglo-Saxon *Netel*, or needle, and may refer to the sharp sting of the plant, but could also be a reference to the fact that the fibers of the Nettle were used to make cloth starting in the 16th century and continuing until as recently as seventy years ago. Nettle fiber is similar to that of hemp or flax and was used for making both very coarse and very fine textured material.

Campbell, a celebrated poet, leaves us these words: "In Scotland, I have eaten nettles. I have slept in nettle sheets and dined off a nettle tablecloth. The young and tender nettle is an excellent potherb and my mother says nettle cloth is more durable than any other species of linen."

German and Austrian scientists agreed with that appraisal and the Nettle was used in the manufacture of army clothing with great success during World War I when cotton was difficult to secure. In 1916, close to three million kilograms of Nettle were harvested in Germany alone and Austria had great quantities under cultivation also. However, producing Nettle cloth by hand as was done in medieval times turned out to be more effective than modern methods. Separating the fibers on a mass production basis with mechanical means proved too difficult to be cost-efficient.

As a healing herb of ages past, Stinging Nettle was so highly regarded that the artist A. Duerer (1471-1528) represented an angel ascending to heaven with a bunch of what is clearly Stinging Nettles clasped in his hands!

An early herbal recommended fresh Nettle juice (or the tincture) as being "of much power inwardly for bleeding from the lungs or stomach" and a small piece of lint, soaked in the juice and placed in the nostril was said to arrest even a severe nose-bleed. Surviving country recipes show that Nettles were often made into a fermented beer much favored by the old folks as a pain reliever for gout and 'the rheumatiz.' Nettle tea is known as a blood purifier and is an important ingredient of many spring tonics around the world.

DESCRIPTION & GROWING REQUIREMENTS: The Stinging Nettle is so familiar it hardly requires an introduction. This perennial grows to a height of two to three feet and is covered with stinging hairs. When brushed against, the sting enters the skin causing great burning and irritation. The drooping green leaves of the Nettle are somewhat heart-shaped and its flowers are the same green and appear in branched clusters springing from the axils of the leaves. Nettles like a good rich, loamy soil with a high degree of moisture.

HOW TO HARVEST & STORE: Wear gloves! The entire plant is a powerful medicinal, including the root, and should be harvested when in flower. The Nettle flowers from late spring to early fall and, as farmers know, are difficult to completely exterminate. Do not fear to dig them from the ground in their entirety so as to bring home your prize, root and all.

Without removing your gloves, tie small bunches of the Nettles together and hang upside down in a warm airy place to dry thoroughly.

When completely dry, break into suitably-sized pieces and store in tightly closed airtight jars. Nettles seem to draw moisture from the air otherwise.

LEGENDARY CURES: The Stinging Nettle has such wide-ranging properties it benefits many different conditions. From Europe, we hear of Nettle tea almost miraculously healing both severe headaches and long-standing eczema in the very busy and bad-tempered mother of seven children. Once her headaches and eczema had eased, she became cheerful and happy and capable of withstanding the tension of attending to her brood.

In another case, an elderly man suffering constant agonizing and apparently medically untreatable headaches was reportedly close to suicide when he began drinking two quarts of Nettle tea every day in desperation. After just four days, he was free of pain and pronounced the Stinging Nettle cure quite incredible!

A middle-aged European woman had a long-standing supperating ulcer high on one cheek-bone which disfigured her otherwise pleasant face and which had caused her almost unbearable pain for over twenty years. She feared the recommended operation and refused to submit to it, causing her doctor a great deal of worry. She writes, "After exactly two weeks, the ulcer had disappeared and I was without pain and it has stayed this way." What effected this miracle-cure? We hear the woman took three cups of Nettle tea with 1 teaspoon of Swedish Bitters (see Chapter 30) added daily.

Even more miraculous is the case of a feeble woman of more than 70 years who was diagnosed as having a number of fatal cancerous growths in her abdomen. Because of her advanced years and generally poor health, her physician felt she could not withstand the necessary operation. A kindly neighbor suggested she take Stinging Nettle tea and she began sipping the infusion throughout the day. After a few months, she went to the doctor for her regular check-up and he expressed amazement. The growths had quite disappeared and the women was more vigorous than she had been in years!

Note: Many respected European herbalists regard the Stinging Nettle as a possible cancer-preventive. It is said that regular long-term ingestion of Stinging Nettle tea prevents any malignancy from finding a favorable environment in the body.

TRADITIONAL USE - INTERNALLY: Along with the properties illustrated in the stories related above, the Stinging Nettle has long been considered a superlative blood-cleansing and blood- building aid. It assists in lowering abnormal blood sugar by stimulating the pancreas and may be of help in cases of hypoglycemia, hyperglycemia and diabetes.

As a gentle diuretic, Stinging Nettle promotes a copious flow of urine and soothes an inflamed urinary tract. With its documented content of iron, Stinging Nettle aids in cases of anemia, chlorosis, and other blood disorders, eliminating the feeling of chronic fatigue and exhaustion. There are those herbalists who insist Stinging Nettle may even be effective against leukemia.

If you suffer from allergies, hay fever and asthma and have a tendency to come down with a cold often, try Stinging Nettle. It is reported to have given the most amazing protection against these afflictions.

Traditionalists insist there is no better 'spring tonic' than the Stinging Nettle. The accepted course of treatment is to prepare a tea from the new spring shoots as they appear and take 1 cupful (without sweetening of any kind) 30 minutes before breakfast and sip an additional 2 cups during the day. Individuals who religiously follow this schedule for four weeks report they feel renewed and refreshed. Hint: If you find the tea unpleasant, add a bit of Mint or Chamomile as flavoring.

This four-week treatment also is suggested for liver complaints of all kinds, gall bladder trouble, stomach cramps, ulcers and any congestion of the respiratory passages. Stinging Nettle is also thought beneficial against virus, fungus and bacterial infections.

TRADITIONAL USE - EXTERNALLY: The rheumatic and arthritic may be relieved of pain by bathing and massaging with Stinging Nettle infusions. Sciatica yields to the Nettle and vascular constrictions caused by sluggish circulation are benefited by the same method.

A tincture of Stinging Nettle is a traditional remedy against unsightly dandruff when regularly massaged into the scalp. Individuals with thinning and falling hair have been helped by using the Stinging Nettle infusion as a hair rinse. Users report the hair comes in thicker in just a few weeks and they no longer find quantities of hair in comb and brush.

HOW TO PREPARE STINGING NETTLE INFUSION (TEA): Pour 6 ounces of freshly boiled water over 1 heaping teaspoon of the herb. Cover and steep for three minutes. Strain and sip unsweetened. Chamomile or mint may be added to improve the taste.

HOW TO PREPARE STINGING NETTLE TINCTURE: Scrub several roots well under cold running water with a stiff brush. Chop finely and place in a glass bottle. Add spirits to cover and leave the bottle undisturbed in a warm place for two week.

HOW TO PREPARE A STINGING NETTLE WASH: Soak 1 heaping handful of scrubbed and chopped root and 2 heaping handfuls of chopped stems and leaves overnight in 5 quarts of cold water. The following day, bring the mixture to a boil, strain and bottle. The wash may be used up to three times before losing all properties.

HOW TO PREPARE NETTLE HAIR RINSE: Bring slowly to a boil 10 heaping handfuls of Nettle parts (fresh or dried) in 5 quarts of water. Remove from heat, cover and steep for six minutes. Cool and strain off the residue.

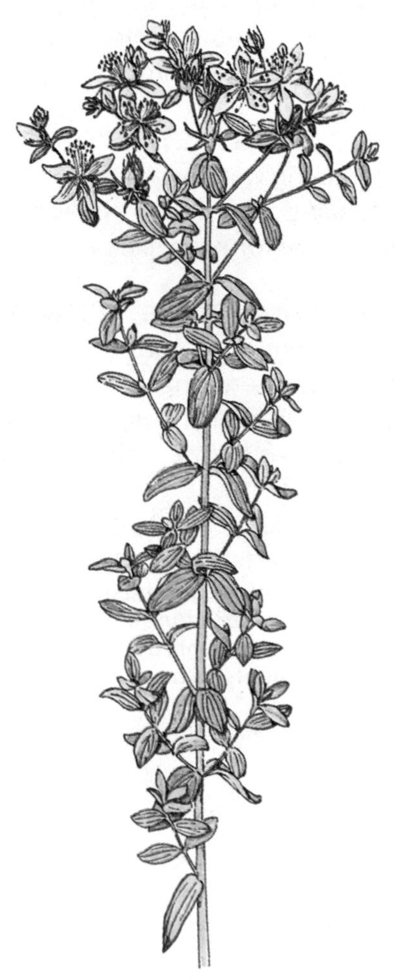

St. John's Wort

Hypericum perforatum

Chapter 30
ST. JOHN'S WORT
(Hypericum perforatum)

Arthritis
Back Pain
Bedwetting
Bruises/Contusions
Colds
Depression
Glands (swollen)
Hysterics
Lumbago
Lymph Glands
Muscles (inflamed)
Muscles (pulled)
Nerve Injury
Nervous Complaints
Neuralgia
Neuritis
Neurosis
Overwork
Restless Sleepers
Rheumatism
Sciatica
Sleepwalking
Speech Disorders
Sprains
Stress
Trigeminal Neuralgia

PAST HISTORY: The bright red oil contained in the leaves of St. John's Wort have been likened to both the blood and wounds of Jesus Christ and to St. John's blood, although this red oil has been called 'Mary's sweat' by country-folk in some locales.

The characteristic spots on the leaves gave rise to the botanical name 'perforatum,' referring to the fact that these spots resemble holes, but are actually subsurface oil glands.

However, most Christian legends dedicate this herb to St. John the Baptist. In medieval times, maidens wore garlands of St. John's Wort twisted around their waists as they danced around bonfires in celebration of St. John's birthday. Branches of the herbs were thrown into the lake to shows the maidens in some mysterious way the suitor they would marry.

The religious connection with this herb is clear, no matter to whom it was dedicated. Branches of the herb and St. John's Wort oil were used to exorcise demons by priests of many early sects.

A charming European custom of ages past was practiced by many farmers who made a sandwich of chopped St. John's Wort and fed it to their barnyard animals to protect them against disease.

DESCRIPTION & GROWING REQUIREMENTS: St. John's Wort is a perennial which grows to a height of one to three feet. This pretty herb bears many branches with yellow-gold flowers and black-spotted leaves. If you are lucky enough to find it growing wild along the roads, in meadows, pastures and woodlands, bring home one or two and it will reward you with both beauty and its medicinal properties.

HOW TO HARVEST & STORE: The entire herb when in flower is harvested for infusions and baths and the newly-opened flowers and leaves for preparation of St. John's Wort oil. Its volatile oils are most potent when the sun is bright and hot, so plan your gathering for midday.

St. John's Wort is best used in fresh form and the infusion may be quick-frozen in ice-cube trays and held for future use in a tightly closed freezer bags. At the close of the chapter, you will find directions for preparing the traditional oil and a tincture, both of which are easily stored.

LEGENDARY CURES: St. John's Wort oil is particularly beneficial in all cases of muscle inflammation as it soothes and heals. A very young child of six, Kathy K., who was diagnosed by her doctor as having a chronic swelling of the lymphatic glands every time she came down with a cold or other childhood complaint, suffered much pain when the condition came upon her.

Kathy's grandmother made up some St. John's Wort oil and rubbed the child's abdomen whenever she doubled up with pain. The glandular swelling was eased and the child was soon up playing happily again. From all reports, this appears to be a permanent cure of her lymphatic involvement.

TRADITIONAL USE - INTERNALLY: St. John's Wort tea is beneficial for all conditions arising from a nerve injury, such as a blow or fall, and nervous afflictions caused by overwork and stress. All nervous complaints, including neuritis, neurosis, and even trigeminal neuralgia (a painful involvement of the 5th cranial nerve), yield to two or three cups daily of St. John's Wort tea sipped hot. In these conditions, a few teaspoons daily of the tincture is particularly beneficial. This treatment should be accompanied by a brisk massage of the affected parts with the oil.

Unfortunate individuals, young or very aged, who suffer the embarrassment of wetting the bed, those who sleep-walk or are restless sleepers, perhaps have a speech disorder, and those who suffer from depression or even have hysterics from time to time, particularly benefit from taking St. John's Wort tea regularly. Along with taking the tea, additional treatment with baths is strongly recommended.

TRADITIONAL USE - EXTERNALLY: For the nervous complaints described above and all nervous complaints in general, the course of treatment with baths is as follows: The affected individual should take one sitz bath, and then foot-baths lasting for a good twenty minutes on the six days following. The soothing and healing effect of these baths greatly potentiates the internal taking of the tea.

St. John's Wort oil is very easily prepared and keeps its potency and healing properties for up to two years. This oil is very effective used as a massage for lower back pain, lumbago, rheumatism, arthritis and sciatica. Contusions, sprains, swollen glands and a pulled muscle will heal more rapidly when the oil is used as a rub. The gentle effect of the oil makes it especially suitable for babies and the very old.

HOW TO PREPARE ST. JOHN'S WORT INFUSION (TEA): Pour 6 ounces of freshly boiled water over 1 heaping teaspoon of the herb. Cover and steep for three minutes. Strain and sweeten with honey, if desired.

HOW TO PREPARE ST. JOHN'S WORT OIL: Gather a quantity of fresh flowers and leaves. Place loosely in a glass bottle and pour in enough cold-pressed olive oil to cover. Cork tightly and allow the to remain undisturbed in a warm place until the oil turns a beautiful red, approximately three to four weeks. Strain the oil through cheesecloth and store in a dark bottle away from light.

HOW TO PREPARE ST. JOHN'S WORT TINCTURE: Place a double handful of freshly picked flowers in a glass bottle. Add enough spirits to cover and place the bottle in a warm place for at least three weeks.

HOW TO PREPARE A ST. JOHN'S WORT BATH: Gather a bucketful of the whole herb, flowers, leaves and stems. Cut coarsely and steep in cold water overnight. The following day, boil briskly, strain, and allow to cool to a comfortable temperature. Use a suitable quantity as an addition to a sitz bath or foot bath.

Chapter 31

SAMST'S SWEDISH BITTERS

PAST HISTORY: If you are not acquainted with the writings of the eminent and greatly respected Swedish physician, Dr. Samst, don't be surprised. Although Dr. Samst's Swedish Bitters have worked the most miraculous cures abroad, Swedish Bitters are little-known in the United States. In fact, very few practicing naturopaths and herbalists in this country are even aware of Swedish Bitters. Among those who have heard of this amazing natural herbal remedy, even fewer know the exact method of preparation.

It is said that regular use of Swedish Bitters may be likened to drinking from the fabled 'Fountain of Youth' in that it apparently assures a lengthened age-span to the ingestor. The author of this wonderful herbal potion, Dr. Samst, lived a long, vigorous and healthy life. Those who were privileged to know the great man during his lifetime say that if he had not died in an accident at the ripe old age of 104 years, he might have lived for 150 years or even longer!

LEGENDARY CURES: A young child of seven years, Timmy H., was severely bitten and deeply scratched on the face by a large alley cat. The child's wounds healed, but left ugly, red welts and deep scars. Following the directions penned by Dr. Samst in what has come to be known as the Old Manuscript, the parents kept the scars and welts well moistened with Swedish Bitters and after a month, the scars did indeed begin to fade away. After six or seven months, Timmy's face was clear.

A Czech refugee, Jan B., who contracted typhoid fever from eating contaminated meat in a refugee camp recovered after being hospitalized when the camp was liberated. But the side-effects of an intestinal obstruction, jaundice, vomiting and diarrhea threatened to put him back in the hospital until he was given some Swedish Bitters. Jan B.'s wife, Elena, made him a compress of Swedish Bitters and wrapped it warmly around his abdomen. Jan said a heat spread through his body which felt as if it swept everything unclean from him. The single compress so relieved his condition that he never again suffered a single symptom.

Martha M., a middle-aged woman of fifty-three years, was continually plagued by a chronic sinus condition which all but incapacitated her. She suffered throbbing headaches and was unable to breathe through her nose at all. Her doctor was talking about doing an operation as a 'last resort' to correct the condition when Mrs. M. discovered Swedish Bitters. For three nights, she slept with a compress of Swedish Bitters applied to her forehead, eyes and nose. On the fourth day, her sinus infection broke and incredible amounts of pus came pouring out her nostrils.

Taking one tablespoon of Swedish Bitters three times daily in herb tea effected an astonishing cure for Georgia N., a pretty young woman who was crippled and lame. Georgia got around painfully with the aid of crutches, but her legs were all but useless. This condition came upon her "overnight," she said, after the birth of her first child, possibly as a result of some unexplainable and unpredictable reaction to the anesthetic. Sadly, her doctors were unable to do anything for her but medicate for the pain.

Georgia finally put her faith in Swedish Bitters and stubbornly persisted, gaining strength as her twisted limbs began every so slowly to return to normal. After eight full months, she was able to discard the crutches and walk with a cane. You can imagine her joy when a year later, Georgia's cure was complete and she could finally romp with her child!

Nettie B., an elderly woman of eighty-three suffered a gradual loss of hearing until she lived in almost a soundless world. Mrs. B. was given a small bottle of Swedish Bitters and, as suggested in the Old Manuscript, began dipping her finger in the drops and then in her ears to moisten the ducts. Before going to bed, she smoothed some Swedish Bitters across her forehead, temples and around the eyes and also put a drop of oil in her ears to counteract the drying effect of the Swedish Bitters. Nettie noticed that gradually her hearing began improving. Within months, she found she was able to enjoy television and could hear and reply to normal conversation. A happy side-effect of her treatment was a fresher, more youthful look to her skin.

TRADITIONAL USE: INTERPRETATION OF THE 'OLD MANUSCRIPT'

Dr. Samst's 'Old Manuscript' lists many uses for Swedish Bitters against as many different conditions of ill health. Most address the problems that can come upon us all - man, woman or child - but some are particularly for female complaints and some are for childhood illnesses.

1. *Alcoholism* - GENERAL: It is written a drunk will become sober immediately by taking two tablespoons of Swedish Bitters diluted in a little cool water.

2. *Anemia* - GENERAL: Swedish Bitters will cleanse the toxins from the blood, aid in forming new blood, stimulate circulation and bring back color to the cheeks if taken regularly every morning for a goodly period of time.

3. *Bruises* - GENERAL: Bruises and painful swellings caused by a blow or a fall quickly yield to a Swedish Bitters compress.

4. *Burns* - GENERAL: Whether they be caused by fire, fat or hot water, burns and scalds are healed if moistened well and often with Swedish Bitters, The Old Manuscript says no blisters will form, the skin is cooled and even infected blisters heal without scarring.

5. *Corns* - GENERAL: Painful corns can be eliminated by applying a cotton ball well moistened with Swedish Bitters to the spot. After three days, the corn will either fall out or can be removed without pain.

6. *Digestive Tract* - GENERAL: It is written that regular use of Swedish Bitters will remedy all troubles of the stomach and intestines, rid the body of gas, aid the liver and regulate the bowels.

7. *Dizziness* - GENERAL: Dizziness and indispositions of all kinds are reputed to yield to regular use of Swedish Bitters, as does lameness.

8. *Ears* - GENERAL: If a piece of cotton be well moistened with Swedish Bitters and put into the affected ear, the pain of an earache will be eased and ringing, buzzing and ear-noises of unknown cause will be eliminated. It is written that Swedish Bitters may restore lost hearing as well.

9. *Erysipelas* - GENERAL: It is written that Erysipelas, a type of streptococcus infection, will yield to regular use of Swedish Bitters.

10. *Eyes* - GENERAL: If the corners of the eyes be moistened with Swedish Bitters, or a moistened cloth be placed over the closed lids, dim, strained eyes become bright and clear and are rid of spots and cataracts. This treatment also works well for inflamed and reddened eyes.

11. *Fever* - GENERAL: An abnormal body temperature, high or low, will be stabilized by taking one tablespoon of Swedish Bitters in hot herb tea. The patient will be strengthened, his pulse will become regular once again and he will soon be healed.

12. *Fistulas* - GENERAL: No matter how old, Swedish Bitters will remedy all fistulas (an abscess or supperating inflammation), even if thought incurable.

13. *Fluid Retention* - GENERAL: For dropsy, edema, bloat and abnormal fluid retention, Swedish Bitters proves to be an effective diuretic if one tablespoon in white wine be taken morning and evening for a period of six weeks.

14. *Frostbite* - GENERAL: A Swedish Bitters compress, kept well moistened, is reputed to heal frostbitten extremities, even if they be open, when applied to the affected parts overnight.

15. *Gall Bladder* - GENERAL: It is written that a painful gall bladder condition may be eased if one tablespoon of Swedish Bitters be taken morning and evening and a compress be applied in the area of the pain and wrapped warmly overnight.

16. *Head* - GENERAL: According to the Old Manuscript, Swedish Bitters will take away headaches, eliminate dizziness, aid the brain and strengthen memory if the vapors are inhaled, the base of the skull moistened with the drops and a well-moistened cloth applied to the head.

17. *Hemorrhoids* - GENERAL: To relieve the pain, itching and burning of hemorrhoids, soak a cotton ball in Swedish Bitters and apply directly to the affected area. Hemorrhoids may be shrunk and softened if Swedish Bitters are taken internally before retiring.

18. *Infectious Diseases* - GENERAL: Swedish Bitters should be taken regularly against plague and other infectious diseases. The drops are reputed to remedy boils and swelling, even if the throat be affected.

19. *Insomnia* - GENERAL: Swedish Bitters taken in hot herb tea before retiring will bring the insomniac a deep, dreamless sleep. The nervous sleeper will find rest by applying a cloth, well-moistened with Swedish Bitters diluted with a little cool water, on the chest overnight.

20. *Joint Pain* - GENERAL: Dr. Samst's Old Manuscript says that when Swedish Bitters are taken morning and evening and a compress is applied to the affected parts, the aches and pains of arthritis, bursitis and rheumatism are eased.

21. *Kidneys* - GENERAL: Kidney conditions are reputed to yield to regular use of Swedish Bitters. As excess fluid in the tissues is eliminated, both appetite and digestion improve. Note: Because the kidneys were thought to be the seat of emotion in the last century, the Old Manuscript states that melancholia and depression will be conquered as well as the kidney condition.

22. *Liver* - GENERAL: Liver complaints, including jaundice, are remedied by taking one tablespoon of Swedish Bitters thrice daily in hot herb tea. For a swollen liver, Dr. Samst says that a Swedish Bitters compress should be applied to the affected area.

23. *Muscle Cramps* - GENERAL: Swedish Bitters are reputed to conquer muscle spasms of all kinds and regular use of the drops will prevent their return.

24. *Scars* - GENERAL: No matter how old or deep, it is written that unsightly scars (even pock marks) will fade away and disappear if moistened constantly with Swedish Bitters for six weeks.

25. *Skin* - GENERAL: Skin rashes, dermatitis, eczema, scabs and pimples heal without scarring if they are moistened regularly with drops of Swedish Bitters.

26. *Stomach Cramps* - GENERAL: Take one tablespoon of Swedish Bitters diluted in a little cool water to eliminate stomach cramps.

27. *Stomach* - GENERAL: Swedish Bitters are highly recommended for nausea, imperfect digestion and all stomach disorders.

28. *Taste (Loss of)* - GENERAL: A loss of the sense of taste (often caused by a vitamin/mineral deficiency in the diet) usually results in a loss of appetite as well. Swedish Bitters are said to bring back the appetite.

29. *Throat* - GENERAL: A sore, inflamed throat which makes it difficult to swallow can be conquered by allowing diluted Swedish Bitters to trickle down the throat thrice daily. This treatment is reputed to cool and heal the condition.

30. *Tongue* - GENERAL: Canker sores, blisters or other complaints of the tongue are said to yield to Swedish Bitters when the drops are frequently applied.

31. *Toothache* - GENERAL: For a toothache or infected gum, hold diluted Swedish Bitters within the mouth on the painful tooth or affected gum area. The infection will heal and the pain will disappear.

32. *Trembling (Palsy)* - GENERAL: The regular ingestion of Swedish Bitters diluted in herb tea or a little water every morning and every evening is said to conquer the trembling of hands and feet.

33. *Warts* - GENERAL: Warts, severely chapped hands and skin cancer are said to yield to Swedish Bitters if the area is kept well moistened with the drops for a period of time.

34. *Wounds* - GENERAL: A new wound should be treated immediately with a compress of Swedish Bitters so that no infection will develop. Wounds that are infected or old wounds which refuse to heal may be remedied by first washing the affected area with white wine and then applying a cloth moistened with Swedish Bitters. They will then heal cleanly without scarring.

35. *Birth (Easy)* - WOMEN: To promote an easy delivery, the pregnant woman is directed to take one tablespoon of Swedish Bitters diluted in cool water every morning and evening for the last fourteen days of pregnancy. To insure that the afterbirth is expelled without pain or complications, one teaspoon of Swedish Bitters should be given every two hours.

36. *Menstruation (Abnormal)* - WOMEN: An abnormal menstrual flow, heavy or light, can be corrected by taking Swedish Bitters for the first three days of the menses. The treatment must be repeated twenty times.

37. *Morning Sickness* - WOMEN: A pregnant woman afflicted with nausea is directed to take one tablespoon of Swedish Bitters in red wine every morning on arising, for three days. After half an hour, a leisurely stroll in the fresh air is recommended before breakfast, which should not include milk. Milk should not be taken with Swedish Bitters.

38. *Nursing Mother* - WOMEN: A nursing mother who suffers swollen, inflammed breasts as the milk dries up will find quick relief if a cloth well moistened with diluted Swedish Bitters be applied to the painful area.

39. *Vaginitis* - WOMEN: A common vaginal discharge with accompanying itching and irritation is said to yield to Swedish Bitters.

40. *Colic* - CHILDREN: A fretful child suffering the pains of colic will quickly be relieved if three tablespoons of well diluted Swedish Bitters are given slowly.

41. *Acne* - TEENS: Swedish Bitters should be taken internally, diluted to suit the age of the individual, and all pimples and pustulas should be moistened frequently with Swedish Bitters as they dry up to prevent scarring.

HOW TO PREPARE DR. SAMST'S SWEDISH BITTERS

Assemble the following ingredients:

2 grams	Saffron
5 grams	Carline Thistle roots
5 grams	Myrrh
10 grams	Aloe*
10 grams	Senna leaves
10 grams	Camphor**
10 grams	Rhubarb roots
10 grams	Zedvoary roots
10 grams	Manna
10 grams	Theriac venezian
10 grams	Angelica roots

* Wormwood powder may be substituted for Aloe
** Natural Chinese Camphor must be used

Put the entire quantity of blended herbs in a 2-quart glass (not plastic) bottle and add 1-1/2 quarts pure spirits to fill the bottle. Cork and allow the bottle to stand in a warm place for two weeks. Shake daily. At the end of the period, strain off the liquid and pour into small bottles. Protect from light and keep tightly corked in a cool place. Shake well before using.
Note: Swedish Bitters becomes more potent the longer it stands.

According to the Old Manuscript, it is written that he who takes Swedish Bitters mornings and evenings daily needs no further medication. Swedish Bitters are a tonic for the nerves and blood, strengthen the body and are reputed to take away all illness. The healing power of Swedish Bitters is said to be so great that it is effective as the basis for every treatment of every illness.
Note: Swedish Bitters should not be taken directly from the bottle, but must always be diluted in water or herb tea.

HOW TO PREPARE SWEDISH BITTERS TO BE TAKEN INTERNALLY: Take Swedish Bitters according to the suggestions in the Old Manuscript as follows: **Morning and evening** - 1 teaspoon Swedish Bitters diluted in a little cool water. **Indispositions of any kind** - up to 3 tablespoons Swedish Bitters diluted in a little cool water may be taken daily. **Serious Complaints** - up to three tablespoons Swedish Bitters may be taken per day. Add 1 tablespoon to a cup of herb tea. Sip half a cup thirty minutes before a meal and the other half thirty minutes after the meal.

HOW TO PREPARE A SWEDISH BITTERS COMPRESS: Because Swedish Bitters is strongly astringent, *protect the skin* by first coating with Calendula ointment (see Chapter 5) or pure lard (not vegetable shortening). Soak a suitably sized piece of sterile gauze in Swedish Bitters and apply to the affected area. Cover the moist cloth with a piece of plastic (such as Saran Wrap), and wrap loosely with soft cloth to hold in the warmth. Allow to remain in place for two to four hours. If the patient can tolerate it, the compress may remain on overnight. Once the compress has been removed, lightly powder the skin to prevent irritation.
Note: If the patient develops a skin rash, omit the compress or use it only for about thirty minutes at a time. If a rash does occur, it may be effectively treated with Calendula ointment.

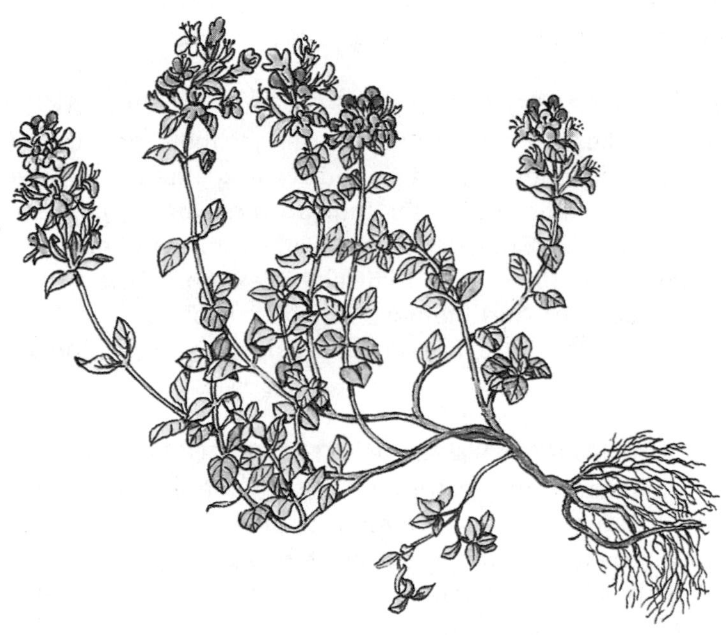

Thyme, Wild

Thymus serpyllum

Chapter 32
THYME, WILD
(Thymus serpyllum)

Alcoholism
Appetite (weak)
Asthma
Bronchitis
Childbirth
Children (hyperactive)
Children (weak)
Colds
Coughs
Depression
Detoxifier
Diuretic
Energizer
Headaches
Epilepsy
Insomnia
Laxative (mild)
Leprosy
Lungs
Menstruation (scanty)
Miscarriage
Multiple Sclerosis
Muscles (taut)
Muscles (weak)
Nervous Complaints
Neuralgia
Phlegm (tough)
Pneumonia
Respiratory Problems
Urine (suppressed)
Whooping Cough

PAST HISTORY: Both Wild Thyme and Garden Thyme (Thymus vulgaris) offer the same medicinal properties. The botanical name for Wild Thyme, *serpyllum,* comes from the Greek and means 'to creep,' descriptive of its growing habits. Wherever this herb grows wild is said to have a singularly pure atmosphere and to enliven the spirits of all who walk near it with its fragrance. The ancient Romans regarded Thyme as the 'sovereign remedy for melancholia' and used it to flavor both cheeses and liqueurs.

It was the cultivated Greeks who dubbed the herb 'Thyme,' a derivative of the Greek word for 'to fumigate,' most likely because it was used as an incense to perfume the air. The high-born Greeks of the day were pleased to be described as 'smelling of thyme.' In medieval England, Thyme was considered a choice strewing herb and was used to cushion dank castle floors where its aromatic scent served to mask the stale body odors of those who bathed infrequently, if at all.

The master herbalist, Culpepper, says Thyme is: "A noble strengthener of the lungs, as notable a one as grows, nor is there a better remedy for hooping cough. It purgeth the body of phlegm and is an excellent remedy for shortness of breath. An oil made of it takes away hot swellings and warts, helps the sciatica and takes away pains and hardness of the spleen. It is excellent for those troubled by the gout and this herb taken inwardly is of great comfort to the stomach."

DESCRIPTION & GROWING REQUIREMENTS: Thyme grows wild very happily in poor soil and basks in sun and heat. As a garden plant, it is very suitable for a rock garden and seems to enjoy the heat radiating from the rocks around it. The dense purple flowers do indeed perfume the air.

This small bedding herb is easily cultivated as long as the soil is light. It despises heavy, rich soil and you would do well to spade in gravel or sand before placing the seed or setting out the clumps.

HOW TO HARVEST & STORE: Thyme flowers profusely from late spring almost until the beginning of autumn. Harvest the mature flowering plant in full sun when the oils are free-flowing and most potent. Dry the clumps of flowers by placing them on a screen in a warm airy place.

LEGENDARY CURES: Since ancient times, sachets of Thyme have been tucked into chests to freshen wearing apparel and herb pillows, with Thyme as the major ingredient, have soothed away headaches and eased the pains of neuralgia.

Thyme's almost magical powers are best illustrated in the story of an old farmer, Hiram B., who was afflicted with a particularly severe form of facial neuralgia for close to thirty years. The poor man's face was out of shape, with his mouth twisted and pulled toward his ear on the right side. Along with the pain, his mouth was permanently open and he had difficulty properly chewing his food.

Only when he began taking Thyme tea regularly and began sleeping on a Thyme pillow his wife made for him did he find relief. After a period of time, the relaxing action of the Thyme eased the taut muscles and his neuralgia was conquered.

The strengthening properties of a Thyme bath are well represented in the tale of a young four-year old child who simply never regained his appetite and former childhood vigor after a long and serious illness. He was pale and wan and no longer wanted to romp with his brothers and sisters, but was content to watch television constantly.

The parents tried many things without success and finally hit upon the idea of a Thyme bath. You can imagine their joy and delight when, after a thirty-minute full soak, the child said he was hungry and wanted to go out and play!

TRADITIONAL USE - INTERNALLY: One of the oldest Herbals says, "Thyme is pungent and hot. It increases the flow of urine and menstruation and, in normal birth, speeds delivery and heals miscarriages as well. A single draught cleanses the noble internal parts of the body."

The medicinal qualities of Thyme were used against leprosy in days of old and, in more recent times, against paralysis and nervous complaints of all kinds. One teaspoonful of Thyme Honey taken before the three daily meals is said to ward off the common cold. A European herbalist has reported great success in epilepsy by using 2 cupfuls of Thyme tea daily for a period of three weeks, ceasing treatment for a ten day interval, and beginning the cycle again.

As a healing herb for respiratory distress, Thyme is used as an infusion with an equal part of Plantain (see Chapter 23). This combination tea, with lemon and honey, assists in ridding the lungs of phlegm in the case of bronchitis or bronchial asthma and eases the racking of whooping cough as well. To ward off pneumonia, a large swallow of the tea taken hot every hour is traditionally recommended.

Ancient herbalists used Thyme very effectively for drunkenness and modern herbalists agree Thyme infusion helps the chronic alcoholic to kick the habit. The accepted method of preparation is to infuse a large handful of Thyme (fresh or dried) in a quart of boiling water. Steep, covered, for three minutes and pour in a pre-warmed thermos so the tea remains hot. The patient must take 1 tablespoon of the infusion every fifteen minutes. The Thyme induces nausea and vomiting and is both laxative and diuretic. Appetite and thirst increase and the patient feels better when fed. Repeat this cleansing treatment after every bout of drink.

TRADITIONAL USE - EXTERNALLY: Overstimulated and highly nervous individuals or those suffering from depression will be rewarded with restful sleep after a twenty-minute full soak in a very warm Thyme bath. Nervous and hyperactive children are especially soothed with this treatment and weak children are strengthened and restored with regular use.

Tincture of Thyme is valuable when used as a brisk massage aid in all cases of muscle weakness of any kind. Multiple sclerosis victims feel renewed strength, as do sickly children and the aged.

HOW TO PREPARE A THYME INFUSION (TEA): Pour 6 ounces of freshly boiled water over 1 heaping teaspoon of the herb (fresh or dried) and steep, covered, for three or four minutes. Strain and sweeten with honey to taste.

HOW TO PREPARE THYME OIL: Gather a quantity of the mature flowering herb and cut coarsely. Place loosely in a glass bottle and fill to cover with cold-pressed olive oil. Cork tightly and allow the bottle to remain undisturbed in a warm place for at least two weeks.

HOW TO PREPARE A THYME TINCTURE: Gather a quantity of the mature flowering herb, cut coarsely and place loosely in a glass bottle. Pour in spirits to cover. Place the bottle in a warm place for two weeks and allow it to remain undisturbed.

HOW TO PREPARE THYME HONEY: In a heavy crock, layer washed, still wet Thyme with raw sugar and press down firmly. Place several thicknesses of waxed paper over the top and weight down so the layers are compressed. Place the crock in a warm place for three or four weeks. Then strain off the syrupy liquid. Rinse the residue in cold water and add to the syrup. Simmer gently over a low heat until the syrup is a honey-like consistency. Bottle and store refrigerated.

HOW TO PREPARE A THYME PILLOW: Using equal parts of sun-dried Thyme, Chamomile (see Chapter 7) and Yarrow (see Chapter 33), crush and lightly stuff a comfortable size pillow. Be sure to select a dense cloth so the herb parts can't poke through and irritate the patient. This pillow is wonderfully soothing and healing.

Chapter 33
WILLOW-HERB (SMALL FLOWERED) (Epilobium parviflorum)

Bladder Problems	*Kidneys*	*Prostate (hypertrophic)*
Bowels (infected)	*Liver Disorders*	*Prostate (inflamed)*
Cancer (bladder)	*Prostate Complaints*	*Ulcer (stomach)*
Diuretic	*Prostate (enlarged)*	*Urine (suppressed)*

PAST HISTORY: The last known reference to the Small-Flowered Willow-Herb appears in an old German Pharmacopeia dating back to the 1800s. Very few current writings on herbs mention the Small Flowered Willow-Herb in any connection, although you will often find a reference to the bark of the Willow *tree* (Salyx) listed. Please do not confuse the two.

The Willow-Herb family (Epilobium) contains nine species, most of which are rich in tannin and are used principally for their astringent properties. The botanical name of the order, Epilobium, comes from two Greek words, *epi* (upon) and *lobos* (a pod) and refers to the fact that the flowers bloom at the tip of the pod-like seed vessels.

Other members of the Epilobium family which have desirable medicinal qualities are the Mountain Willow-Herb (montanum), the Dark-Green Willow-Herb (obscurum), the Lance-Leafed Willow-Herb (lanzeolatum), the Hill Willow-Herb (collinum), the Marsh Willow-Herb (palustre), the Gravel Willow-Herb (fleischeri) and the Alpine Willow-Herb (anagallidifolium).

DESCRIPTION & GROWING REQUIREMENTS: The valuable Willow-Herbs all have one thing in common, and that is the tiny size of their flowers. Willow-Herb blossoms may be white to pastel-pink to a rusty red hue, but always appear at the tip of the long, thin seed pods. When the seed pods break open, silky white hairs are revealed, fastened onto the tiny seeds. All the Willow-Herbs like a rich, loamy soil and a lot of moisture.

HOW TO HARVEST & STORE: This herb is used in the fresh or dried state. If you wish, once you have prepared the infusion of the fresh

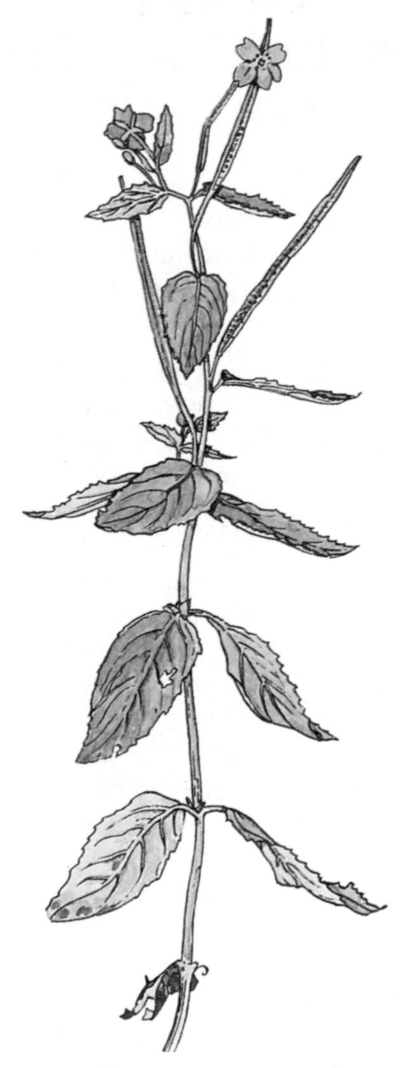

Willow-Herb (Small Flowered)

Epilobium parviflorum

plant, you may freeze a quantity in ice cube trays for later use. Once solidly frozen, place the cubes in a freezer bag and close tightly.

The *small-flowering* varieties listed in the text offer equal medicinal properties and are interchangeable. Do not harvest the entire stem, but take care to pinch it off in the middle in order to allow the plant sufficient growth to put forth new side-shoots. Bring home stems containing both leaves and flowers. Pass by any of the large flowered varieties. They are not used.

LEGENDARY CURES: The files of a renowned European herbalist hold this heart-rending letter from Carl J.: "I beg you to show me a way back to health. Give my family back their healthy father." Mr. J. suffered from a chronic and very painful inflammation of the prostate gland. He passed pus and blood everytime he had a bowel movement and developed a serious liver disorder and a stomach ulcer. The medication he required for his condition had destroyed all his friendly intestinal bacteria, allowing the side conditions to develop. Finally, on doctor's orders, he eliminated all medication.

Mr. J. went through an operation on his prostate, but still the inflammation did not subside and his physician put him back on the original medication and gave him injections to boost the effect. Once again, his condition worsened. If Mr. J. had but known of the Small-Flowered Willow-Herb in time, his many years of suffering might have been unnecessary.

The case of William E. graphically illustrates the tremendous power of the Small-Flowered Willow-Herb. He writes: "The Small-Flowered Willow-Herb has relieved my prostate disorder. I was in the hospital with a heart infarction, but also suffered from prostate disorder. Because of my heart condition, the doctor didn't believe I could withstand an operation. When I heard of the wonderful Willow-Herb which had helped in so many similar cases, I began to drink three cups daily. After several days, I had no more complaints. I still drink two cups daily for a complete recovery. I thank God from the bottom of my heart for the Small-Flowered Willow-Herb. It is unbelievable that medicinal plants give such results!"

In a young woman, Anne K., who had been diagnosed as having cancer of the bladder, the disease had progressed to the point where she was hospitalized and suffering great pain. Miss K.'s doctor allowed the use of the Willow-Herb infusion, but said he was doubtful anything could help. Miss K. drank one cup in the morning and one in the evening for two weeks and found she was actually feeling better at the end of that period. Even the doctor had to admit the herb helped.

TRADITIONAL USE - INTERNALLY: As the stories above clearly show, the Small-Flowered Willow-Herb is of great assistance in any type prostate disorder, including inflammation, enlargement, and even hypertrophy of the gland.

For kidney and bladder dysfunction, the herb's astringent and diuretic properties may bring relief. Cases of suppressed urine often yield to the Willow-Herb.

It must be noted that as all disorders grow and develop over a lengthy period of time, the Willow-Herb tea must be taken regularly over a lengthy period of time for its healing properties to be effective. In even the most severe and serious conditions, only two cups daily should be taken. Ideally, one cup is sipped in the morning on an empty stomach before breakfast and the second cup is taken at least thirty minutes before the last meal of the day.

TRADITIONAL USE - EXTERNALLY: In spite of diligent research, we find no instance where the Small-Flowered Willow-Herb is recommended for external use.

HOW TO PREPARE SMALL-FLOWERED WILLOW-HERB INFUSION (TEA): Using the fresh herb only (stems, leaves, flowers), mince finely a heaping teaspoon for every 6 ounces of freshly boiled water. Cover and steep for three or four minutes and sip hot. It is best not to sweeten this tea.

Chapter 34
YARROW
(Achillea millefolium)

Abdominal Problems	*Colds*	*Menopausal Problems*
Angina Pectoris	*Decongestant*	*Menses (at puberty)*
Appetite (weak)	*Depression*	*Menses (irregular)*
Arthritis	*Digestive Tract*	*Migraines*
Back Pain	*Eyes (tearing)*	*Nausea*
Bedwetting	*Female Complaints*	*Neuritis*
Blood (builder)	*Fibroids*	*Nosebleeds*
Blood (purifier)	*Gas (flatulence)*	*Ovaries (inflamed)*
Bone Marrow	*Headaches*	*Rheumatism*
Bowels (sluggish)	*Hemorrhoids*	*Sinuses (to drain)*
Bursitis	*Intestines*	*Stomach (bleeding)*
Cancer (abdominal)	*Kidneys*	*Stomach (cramps)*
Cancer (lungs)	*Liver*	*Uterus (prolapsed)*
Circulatory Disorders	*Lungs (bleeding)*	*Vaginal Discharge*

PAST HISTORY: This universal herb has been used and appreciated around the world for centuries. Its common name, Yarrow, is thought to be a corruption of the Dutch *yerw*, but may have derived from the Anglo-Saxon term *gearwe*, depending on the source consulted. Yarrow was used in the Scandanavian countries, especially in Norway, as a cure for rheumatism, and the fresh leaves were chewed to stop a toothache. The Swedes called it 'Field Hop' and used it in the place of Hops for brewing beer, as did the Afrikaners. In the Scottish Highlands, country-folk employ Yarrow in an ointment yet today and the tea is famous for curing depression and melancholy no matter what the cause.

Yarrow was one of the herbs used in magic spells during the Middle Ages. One of the old legends says, "If Yarrow be tucked under the pillow and a certain spell be spaked a'fore sleep," the dreamer was promised a 'night vision' (dream) of his or her future mate.

Yarrow's botanical name, *Achillea*, is reputed to refer to the fable that the famed warrior Achilles used it to staunch the bleeding wounds his soldiers suffered in battle. Early common names for Yarrow include

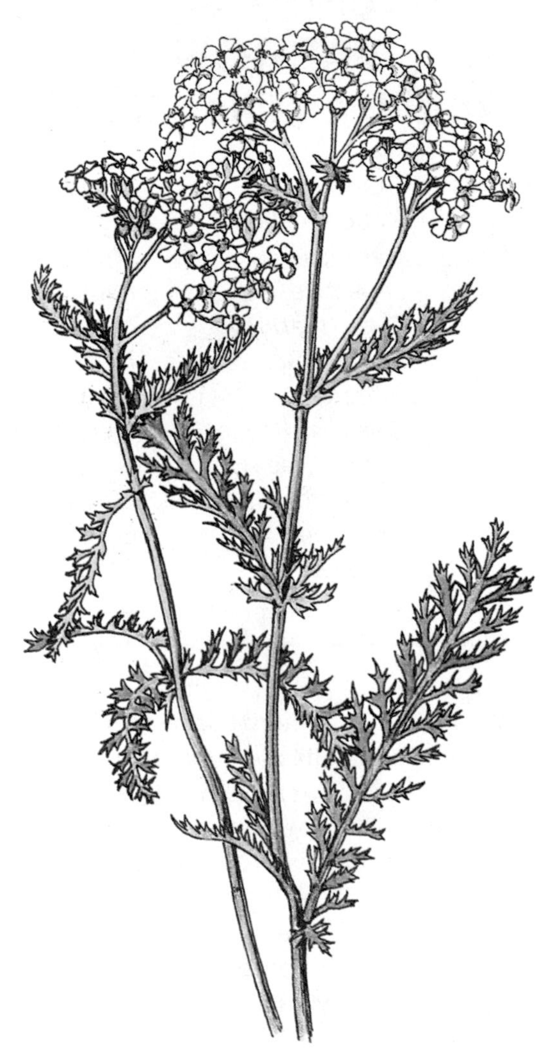

Yarrow

Achillea millefolium

the Soldier's Wound Wort and the Knight's Milfoil and certainly credit the styptic (blood-clotting) properties of the herb.

DESCRIPTION & GROWING REQUIREMENTS: You have probably walked by Yarrow growing wild in meadows and pastures many times without paying it the attention it deserves. This tall herb carries finely toothed leaves which appear almost feathery. The Yarrow is in flower from June to September in most climates and the flower heads of white, palest pink or faint lavender resemble clusters of tiny daisies. Yarrow transplants well and may be grown from seed in just about any type soil, but prefers a sunny location.

HOW TO HARVEST & STORE: The best time to gather Yarrow is to take the mature plant in July or August. Plan your harvesting expedition for around mid-day when the sun-heated plant's volatile oils are free-flowing and most potent. Snip the entire herb, stems, leaves and flowers.

The plant is best used fresh, but you may tie bunches together and hang upside down in a warm airy place to dry for winter use.

LEGENDARY CURES: The tale is told of Susan J., a young woman of 19 who had not yet menstruated. In an effort to bring on her menses, her doctor prescribed birth-control pills. Susan's breasts became larger, a common and not entirely unwelcome side-effect of 'the pill,' but she did not begin menstruating. The girl was tense and depressed and finally refused to continue her medication. An herbalist recommended Susan take one cup of Yarrow tea each morning before breakfast when her stomach was empty. After a month of this treatment, the young lady's system was apparently corrected and her menses began. From all reports, her monthly period is now both regular and normal.

There is no better herb for abdominal complaints than Yarrow, as the following story demonstrates. A fine twenty-eight year old young man by the name of Charles W., husband and father of two children, was diagnosed as having cancer of the abdomen. He was hospitalized, operated upon and had embarked on a course of chemotherapy and cobalt treatments on an out-patient basis, but his physician didn't hold out much hope.

His wife refused to give up on her beloved husband and prepared him Yarrow tea daily, insisting he drink as much as he could hold. Although Mr. W. didn't believe in the medicinal herbs, he drank up to two quarts of the infusion every day just to please his wife. A little over a month later, he was amazed to find the nausea caused by the chemotherapy was easing and he could hold down his food again. Mr. W. began to put on some of the weight he had lost and slowly and surely felt better and better. At last report, Charles W. was continuing to take Yarrow daily and continuing to improve.

TRADITIONAL USE - INTERNALLY: Yarrow is especially valuable for all female complaints. It has been said that women in general could be spared many problems if they would just take Yarrow tea from time to time. Yarrow is noted for promoting the easy and timely onset of the menses in puberty, for regularizing and normalizing an abnormal menstrual flow and for eliminating the usual problems of menopause.

Yarrow tea is a good decongestant and promotes sinus drainage, thereby conquering the pain of a sinus headache. Even migraine headaches have been known to yield to Yarrow. If taken on a regular basis, migraines may be entirely eliminated. Chronic nosebleeds, a pain behind the eyes and even eyes which tear constantly have been helped by regular use of Yarrow.

Yarrow is one of the finest of the blood-cleansing herbs and even acts on bone-marrow and stimulates blood production. For a disorder of the marrow, the tea should be taken and the tincture and sitz baths also employed.

With its astringent and styptic action, Yarrow is thought beneficial for internal stomach bleeding, bleeding hemorrhoids and even bleeding of the lungs. Prominent herbalists recommend Yarrow tea and Calamus root (see Chapter 4) as a remedy in cases of lung cancer. The accepted course of treatment is to take two cups of Yarrow tea (morning and evening on an empty stomach) and chew Calamus root throughout the day.

Yarrow is said to stimulate kidney and gastrointestinal functioning, benefit the liver, encourage the appetite and to dispel gas-causing stomach cramps. Sluggish bowels become normal with the peristaltic stimulating action of Yarrow. The pain and spasms of angina pectoris may be eased by regular use of Yarrow and it is of help in any circulatory disorder as well.

Sipping hot Yarrow tea in great amounts is traditionally recommended for colds, lower back pain and the aches of rheumatism, bursitis and arthritis. For these conditions, a pinch of hot cayenne pepper should be added to increase the warming action of the Yarrow.

TRADITIONAL USE - EXTERNALLY: See text above for suggested use of the tincture. A Yarrow sitz bath is a tremendous aid to general health and well-being. For women in particular, it is said a Yarrow sitz bath often relieves the pain of inflamed ovaries, heals the condition causing a common vaginal discharge (as does a wash) and aids in correcting a prolapsed uterus.

In the case of a prolapsed uterus, a combination treatment is suggested. Along with the Yarrow sitz baths, four cups of Lady's Mantle tea (see Chapter 19) is taken daily and the abdominal area is massaged with a tincture of Shepherd's Purse (see Chapter 26).

A Yarrow sitz bath may be employed against the embarrassing nightly bedwetting of children or the very aged. As a soothing treatment for neuritis, Yarrow baths often relieve pain after just one use. These sitz baths are especially recommended for fibroids and should be continued until the physician pronounces the cure complete.

Yarrow flower ointment relieves the burning and itching of hemorrhoids.

HOW TO PREPARE YARROW TEA: Pour 6 ounces of freshly boiled water over 1 heaping teaspoon of the minced herbs. Cover and steep for three or four minutes. Strain, but do not sweeten. Sip hot.

HOW TO PREPARE A YARROW TINCTURE: Gather a quantity of Yarrow flowers in the hot noonday sun and place loosely in a glass bottle. Fill to cover with spirits. Cork and allow the bottle to remain undisturbed in a warm place for two weeks. Note: This is an excellent method of 'storing' fresh Yarrow. Two tablespoons of the tincture to one cupful of the tea.

HOW TO PREPARE A YARROW BATH: Gather a quantity of fresh Yarrow. Steep a double handful of the snipped flowers, leaves and stems overnight in two quarts of cold water. The following day, bring the blend to a full boil, strain and add to the bath.

HOW TO PREPARE A YARROW OINTMENT: On low heat, liquify 2 cups of pure lard (not vegetable shortening) and add 1/2 cup each fresh Yarrow flowers and Raspberry leaves, both snipped fine. Raise the heat to medium and stir the mixture until it simmers. Remove from heat and allow the blend to stand overnight. The following day, warm to liquify and strain through cheesecloth. Add 2 tablespoons of cold-pressed olive oil to help keep the ointment soft, pour into clean glass jars and refrigerate.

Chapter 35
YELLOW & WHITE DEAD NETTLES
(Lamium galeobdolon & Lamium album)

Abdominal Problems
Bladder (infected)
Digestive Tract
Diuretic
Female Complaints
Insomnia
Kidneys
Kidneys (cirrhosis)
Menstrual Cramps
Nephritis
Skin Conditions
Ulcers
Urine (suppressed)
Varicose Veins

PAST HISTORY: The 'Dead' Nettles earned their name because of their inability to 'sting.' The family bears a close resemblance to the Stinging Nettles and this protective device of Mother Nature makes them as unattractive to browsing animals and leaf-eating insects as the true 'stinging' Nettles.

The botanical name of the Yellow Dead Nettle, 'galeobdolon,' comes from two Greek words, *gale* (weasel) and *bdolos* (an unpleasant odor). Country-folk often call the Yellow Dead Nettle "Weasel Snout" and the herb does have a most unpleasant odor until it has been dried.

The White Dead Nettle is sometimes called "White Archangel," possibly because it flowers close to May 8th, dedicated in the old calendar to the Archangel Michael.

The generic name of the Dead Nettles, 'Lamium,' is from the Greek *laimos,* or throat, and refers to the 'throat-shaped' form of its blossoms. Master Herbalist Culpepper says the Dead Nettles "maketh the heart merry, drive away melancholy, quicken the spirits, stauncheth bleeding at the mouth and nose if they be stamped and applied to the nape of the neck." Ancient herbalists used the dried herb as an infusion to promote perspiration, believing it acts efficaciously on the kidneys.

DESCRIPTION & GROWING REQUIREMENTS: The Dead Nettles are found growing companionably alongside the Stinging Nettles and like a moist, rich, loamy soil in partial shade. The Yellow Dead Nettle

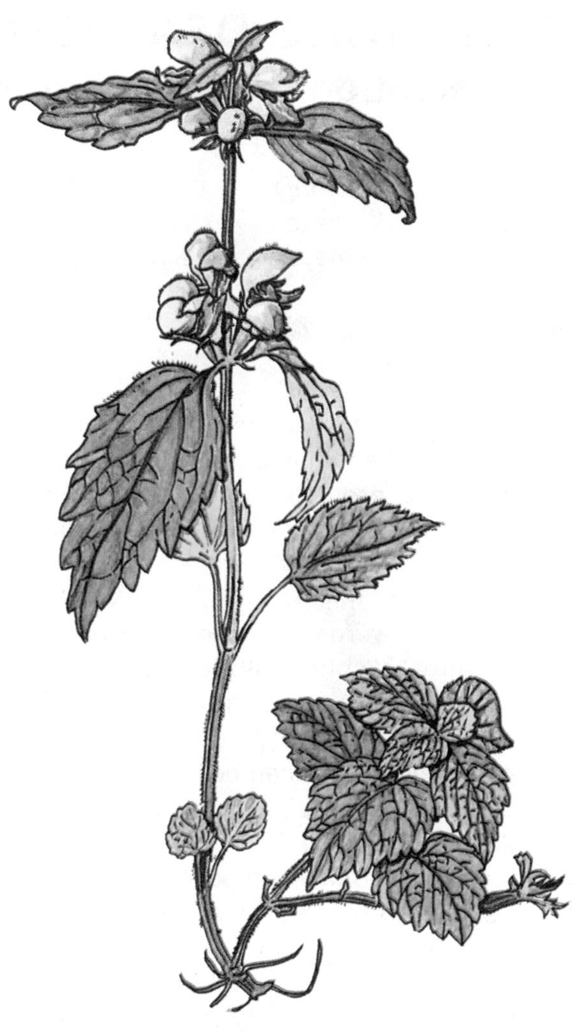

Yellow Dead Nettle

Lamium Galeobdolon

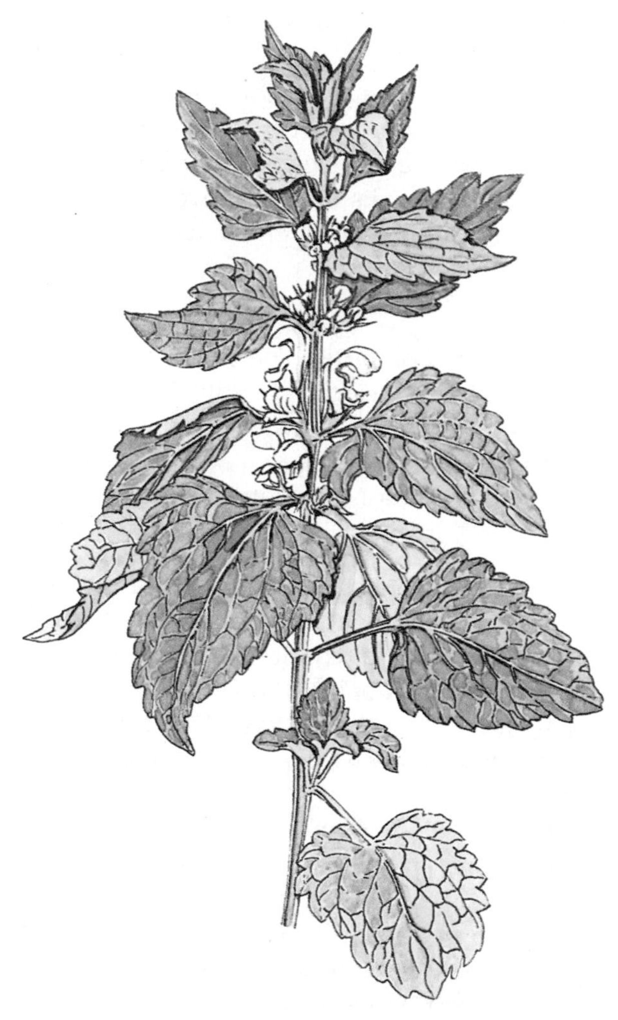

White Dead Nettle

Lamium album

offers us large handsome flowers, yellow with red blotches, for only two months of the year. Its stem stands straight up with pairs of narrow, pointed leaves.

The White Dead Nettle has a much longer blooming season and its creamy-white flowers may be seen from May until autumn in most climates. Both White and Yellow Dead Nettles put forth their blossoms in whorls from amidst the axils of their leaves and both have almost square, hollow stems. Country children often cut the stems and make a whistle out of them.

HOW TO HARVEST & STORE: The properties of these valuable medicinal herbs are almost interchangeable. Both should be gathered as mature flowering plants. Tie the stems together in small bunches and hang upside down in a warm airy place to dry thoroughly. Don't worry - the characteristic odor dissipates as the herbs dry.

LEGENDARY CURES: The Dead Nettles are mildly diuretic and considered beneficial in cases of bladder infection, as this story illustrates: A sixty-three year old gentleman by the name of George H. suffered from a chronic bladder infection that created sharp pain when it was upon him. Mr. H. took the course of antibiotics that his doctor prescribed and all would be well for a time until suddenly the condition would flare up again.

After six months of being on and off medication constantly, Mr. H. became impatient and decided to try the old herbal remedy his neighbor had been after him to take. The neighbor prepared a combination of equal parts of dried Yellow Dead Nettle, Cleavers (see Chapter 8) and Golden Rod (see Chapter 14) and told George H. how to make the tea himself. He followed her directions, taking one cupful of tea in the morning and one again in the evening.

Astonishingly, George H. never developed a bladder infection again. One happy side-effect the neighbor hadn't thought to tell him about was that the insomnia he suffered was apparently cured in the bargain.

TRADITIONAL USE - INTERNALLY: As the preceeding story shows, Yellow Dead Nettle is particularly beneficial in the case of chronic bladder infections, suppressed or burning urine and all cases of bladder malfunction, especially in the elderly. The insomniac often finds dreamless sleep upon taking a cup of Dead Nettle tea before retiring.

Women who dread the onset of their monthly menses because they suffer cramps find relief and many of the so-called 'female complaints' are eased by regular use of the tea as well. In fact, anyone with a chronic digestive or abdominal complaint will benefit from the properties of the Dead Nettles.

Kidney disorders, including nephritis, and even fluid retention with cardiac involvement, may yield to continual use of the Dead Nettle infusions. The cleansing combination of Yellow Dead Nettle, Cleavers and Golden Rod is of particular benefit in cirrhosis of the kidneys, even when the patient is on dialysis.

In the case of non-specific dermatitis (an unidentified skin condition), a single cup of Dead Nettle tea taken on an empty stomach upon arising in the morning has been known to work wonders.

TRADITIONAL USE - EXTERNALLY: A Dead Nettle sitz bath is a useful adjunct to the internal use of the tea in all cases of bladder and kidney involvement and is especially soothing for abdominal complaints of any kind, including menstrual cramps.

A warm Dead Nettle compress quickly eases throbbing and aching varicose veins. The compress is also of benefit for ulcers.

HOW TO PREPARE A DEAD NETTLE INFUSION (TEA): Pour 6 ounces of freshly boiled water over 1 heaping teaspoon of the lightly crushed dried herbs. Cover and steep for three or four minutes. Strain and sip hot.

HOW TO PREPARE DEAD NETTLE COMBINATION TEA: Pour 6 ounces of freshly boiled water over 1 heaping teaspoon of equal parts of a blend of dried Yellow Dead Nettle, Cleavers and Golden Rod. Cover and steep for three or four minutes. Strain and use as directed in the text.

HOW TO PREPARE A DEAD NETTLE SITZ BATH: Soak two double handfuls of the entire dried herb (stems, leaves and flowers) overnight in 2 quarts of fresh cold water. The following morning, bring the mixture to a boil. Cool to a comfortable temperature, strain and add to the sitz bath.

HOW TO PREPARE A DEAD NETTLE COMPRESS: Pour 16 ounces of freshly boiled water over 3 heaping teaspoons of the dried herb. Cover and steep for 10 minutes. Cool slightly. Soak a clean white cloth in the infusion and apply to the affected area. Wrap warmly.

Chapter 36
THE F-M CIRCULIZER SYSTEM
New to the U.S. — European Herbal Therapy

THE HERBAL FOOTBATH: After reading this chapter, you'll become aware of how advanced the overseas medical community is in the use of herbs. We have been searching the world investigating alternative forms of health therapies to bring back to the U.S. In our travels, we discovered a very important herbal treatment that is virtually unknown in America. For over 40 years, health specialists abroad have been using selected herbal essence blends with a temperature-controlled footbath device to *influence the vital blood circulation system* of the body. This is the first introduction of the temperature-controlled herbal footbath system to the American public.

THE F-M SYSTEM

THE UNIT ITSELF: This treatment system consists of a self-contained unit which the user fills with water and a prescribed herbal blend. But the real secret of this incredible device is the precise gradations of temperature that are preprogrammed into it. This clever machine first heats the water to the necessary temperature. Then the device gently raises the temperature of the water very gradually until the full power of the botanical essence has been released, thus insuring absorption of all medicinal properties.

Science has determined that the benefits of the prescribed herbs, when combined with this graduated and precisely controlled rise in temperature, are immeasurably enhanced. Tests have shown that the combination of herbs and the gradual rise in temperature greatly influences the entire circulatory system, the vascular system, and the inner organs of the body as well.

HERE'S HOW IT WORKS: The explanation is simple. In scientific circles, this phenomenon is known as the *'Dastre-Moratsche'* or *'consensual'* reaction. A good example of this reaction is the person who goes walking on a cold winter day. Let us suppose he inadvertently breaks through a thin film of ice covering a stream of almost frozen water which is deep enough to thoroughly soak his boots and the socks beneath. Because he has drastically lowered the temperature of the sensitive thermal receptors on the soles of his feet, he very soon develops a serious head cold. Even though his feet are far removed from the mucous membranes of his nose and sinus cavities, they are affected by this change in temperature. Measurements show that the temperature of the mucous membranes of the velum, oral cavity, and outer auditory canals drops when the feet are cold.

On the other hand, the temperature controlled herbal footbath, its slowly rising temperature, results in a beneficial effect that works by first expanding the tiny capillaries in the soles of the feet. As the temperature rises, the deep-seated larger arterioles and then the big blood vessels of the feet expand. Very soon, all the blood vessels of the feet are expanded to the maximum and this expansion effect travels upwards throughout the entire body, including the head region, carrying with it the medicinal properties of the herbs as they are absorbed.

CIRCULATORY COMPLICATIONS ARE MANY

CONDITIONS BENEFITED: Some of the conditions successfully treated with herbs and the controlled temperature device include: influenza, colds, bronchitis, angina, bladder infections, asthma, migraine headaches, circulation problems, intermittent claudication, high cholesterol and triglyceride levels, rheumatism, dizziness, insomnia, eczema, psoriasis, arthritis, kidney problems, arteriosclerosis, osteoporosis, both high and low blood pressure, senility, varicose veins, glaucoma, hypercalcemia, angina pectoris, heart arrhythmia, impotence, lupus erythematosis, gangrene, prostate problems, and on and on.

Extensive medically-supervised tests show this system to be a revolutionary approach to many health problems related to or complicated by poor circulation. In modern society, poor circulation is a universal problem, even in younger people. Many illnesses are associated with circulatory impairment. Circulatory problems are especially evident with advancing age. This herbal footbath can be used by anyone of any age in the privacy of the home. As an aid to stimulating circulation, it promises to be an effective preventive and prophylactic treatment to assist in overcoming existing illnesses and/or to guard against circulatory complaints.

EMPIRICAL EVIDENCE ABOUNDS

THE TESTIMONIALS POUR IN: If this method of treatment seems too good to be true, read on. From the files of various physicians, comes a wealth of empirical evidence. The results detailed in the following stories of grateful patients will convince you.

Consider the case of Mrs. Marie B., an 84-year-old woman suffering from arthrosis deformans of hip and knee joints. Her condition was subsequently complicated by gall stones, cystitis, and peritonitis. After an emergency operation (at age 82) which resulted in the removal of 8 feet of bowel, Mrs. B. was bedridden. After many months, she was eventually able to drag herself around painfully with the aid of crutches. Thrombosis and an embolism of one lung followed, but still she survived in spite of the fact that her doctors considered her case hopeless.

A series of treatments with the herbal footbath restored this woman almost miraculously. Mrs. B. herself says, "My health is better now than it was 20 years ago and I feel much younger! To me, these herb footbaths are a real Fountain of Youth. All my illnesses have gone. My friends often ask, 'What is it that keeps you young?' I tell them that my blood is circulating again the way it did when I was in my teens and all the impurities that were making me sick have been flushed out of my body by the prescribed herbal blend. This method works excellently and is well worth the cost!"

The treatment of an 83-year old male patient suffering from hypertrophic prostatis, George H., was complicated by a dangerous heart condition that precluded surgery. To further add to Mr. H.'s problem was the fact that the gland had enlarged to the size of a hen's egg. Because even the most weakened heart is not endangered by the therapeutic herbal footbath, this gentleman was started on the baths immediately. After a four-week course of therapy, the enlargement was found to have vanished completely. Mr. H.'s medical doctor confessed to being amazed, so sure was he that the condition would only grow worse.

A 57-year old man who also suffered from an enlarged prostate had borne the condition for ten years before he was introduced to the herbal footbath. Thomas C.'s condition had progressed to the point where he was unable to urinate for some days and his doctor was considering the use of a catheter to afford him relief. Incredibly, just one herbal footbath dissolved the blockage within fifteen minutes. Mr. C. is continuing with therapy to insure that his prostate remains normal.

A registered nurse by the name of Rebecca W. was the victim of terrible headaches caused by a serious frontal sinusitis condition which had plagued her for over ten years. She spoke of feeling as if her eyes were being pulled from their sockets and was terrified because she felt she was going blind. Miss W. says, "These headaches were so violently painful that at times I actually considered suicide to escape the agony."

As a trained nurse, Miss W. was skeptical of the herbal footbath, but agreed to try a series of treatments in what she frankly called "pure desperation." The first few baths brought her no relief, and she had to be persuaded to continue. But after the sixth bath, her infection broke and she began discharging thick globs of pus from both nostrils. This foul-smelling purulent discharge continued for about ten days. After her thirteenth footbath, the discharge disappeared along with her violent headaches. Miss W. says, "I'm a true believer now. In fact, I advised a friend who also suffered from a severe sinus condition to take the baths and she, too, has been completely cured. We are both so thankful. Many people don't understand the agony a chronic sinus infection can cause. It's hard to describe the joy I feel about what this simple therapy has accomplished!"

For over twenty-nine years, a professional man in his mid-fifties had suffered from severe asthma and a serious cardiac weakness. Paul Y. was medically treated with injections for both asthma and his heart. He regularly inhaled a bronchodialator compound in order to breathe comfortably.

Mr. Y.'s condition went from bad to worse. He was being transported via ambulance to a full-care facility when he lapsed into unconsciousness. His heart stopped beating and he was turning blue when a strong injection directly into his heart roused him.

Fortunately, a health care specialist trained in the use of the herbal footbath took an interest in his case. Mr. Y was treated therapeutically with prescribed herbs and the controlled-temperature footbath. After fifteen treatments, his asthma disappeared and his heart complaint was eased to the point where Mr. Y. is once again working at his profession. He now takes precautionary maintenance treatments.

A man of 43 years, Mr. Ludwig F., developed a serious case of scabies and was advised by his doctor to use a prescribed liquid for relief. Mr. F. found that the condition worsened instead of getting better. He was to the point where the only relief he found from the intolerable itching and pain was to scald himself in the shower.

After consulting a naturopathic doctor, Mr. F. used medicinal herbs and the footbath system. Just three days later, the itching began to ease and within a few days, Mr. F. was completely cured.

The herbal footbath was recommended to Mr. John B., 74 years of age, for a kidney condition. As a cigarette smoker for some sixty years of his life, Mr. B.'s circulation was understandably impaired. Although he had been told by many doctors over the years to stop smoking because it was seriously undermining his health, Mr. B. did not do so. At this writing, he has had only two sessions on the bath and it is too early to judge results as they apply to his kidney problem.

However, after just these two herbal bath treatments, Mr. B. reported in amazement that he had lost all desire to smoke and refused a cigarette when it was offered to him! (Note: This system has not been tested as a deterrent to smoking. Without further evidence, we must consider Mr. B.'s testimony as a purely personal statement which applies in his case alone, but we can conjecture that his system was purged of addicting nicotine. His case presents an interesting premise that should be explored further.)

Other grateful patients have written of their experiences using the herbal footbath as well. We include here excerpts from a few letters:

"We are convinced of the good effect of the herbal footbath. My husband is completely cured of the rheumatism that made him miserable for 20 years," N.M.

"I had been suffering with varicose veins for many years and the pain handicapped me greatly. After twenty herbal footbaths, I was completely cured and all complaints connected with my varicose veins are gone. I stand eight hours a day at work, but the varicosities have not returned. I recommend the baths to everyone." B.L.

"As a nineteen-year old girl, I was made very unhappy because my face was disfigured with terrible acne. My doctor told me to eat a lot of fruit, cut down on the fat in my diet, and prescribed some herbs to use with the footbath. I did just what he told me to do." (Note: This young woman had the worst case of acne I have ever seen with eruptions the size of a nickel covering her face and back.) "I was so afraid I'd be scarred for life, but even the deep pits seem to be clearing. After two months, my skin is clear and soft and has a healthy look. I can't tell you what a difference this has made in my life!" S.D.S.

TO STIMULATE CIRCULATION & FLUSH AWAY TOXINS

THE PRESCRIBED HERBAL BLENDS: When used with precisely prescribed medicinal herbs, the controlled-temperature footbath system both improves vital blood circulation and works to flush the toxins out of the body. It is a medical fact that the skin is the largest eliminative organ of the body. Many impurities are excreted through the pores of the skin, carried outside along with the perspiration that helps regulate the temperature of the body. To understand this process, consider the stale smell of an unwashed body. Your nose tells you of the impurities collected on the surface of the skin which need to be washed away.

This premise is confirmed by the use of the herbal footbath. Very often patients undergoing treatment will complain of a sick stench coming from their skin. They should rejoice! There's more room on the outside than there is on the inside. This odor is proof-positive that the impurities and toxins contributing to a condition of ill health are being gradually eliminated. The skin is doing its job superlatively!

Another virtue which must be exercised in the use of the controlled-temperature herbal footbath is that of patience. It is unreasonable to expect immediate results from this natural form of therapy. If you have lived in this polluted and imperfect world for 20, 30, or 50 years, your body has unavoidably been accumulating toxins for 20, 30, or 50 years. When the impurities get stirred up and the healthy red blood begins coursing through your veins again as it did when you were a child, improvement is steady and sure.

For more information on this system, write to:

New Dimensions Distributors
2419 N. Black Canyon Highway, Suite #7
Phoenix, Arizona 85009
Call Toll-Free 1-800-624-7114 — Extension 12
In Arizona Call: (602) 257-1183

Chapter 37
AIDS & ITS HERBAL HELPERS

AIDS, the Acquired Immune Deficiency Syndrome, is spreading across America at a truly alarming rate. Although authorities once thought this dread condition was a threat only to homosexual males, it has become increasingly apparent that other segments of the population are also at risk.

To understand the importance of the body's immune system, we need only to recall those few unfortunate and highly-publicized children who were born without the ability to produce the antibodies necessary for protection against infection and disease. Because even the common cold could become a life-threatening crisis, these children could only be kept alive inside a plastic bubble in a totally sterile, germ-free, artifically-produced atmosphere.

We can't live our lives inside a plastic bubble - and certainly most of us wouldn't want to be so isolated from family and friends anyway. Fortunately, new research indicates that there are certain medicinal herbs that can provide the very elements which have been shown to stimulate and enrich the body's immune defense system.

Are there actually certain cure-all miracle herbs that can help prevent the lethal AIDS virus, which causes such an agonizing slow death, from infiltrating your system? According to many expert and respected authorities, the answer is *yes*.

Dr. James Duke, a botanist associated with the Agriculture Department in Beltsville, Maryland, was quoted as saying, "Herbs are high in vitamin and minerals. That's the key to their success in boosting resistance to disease."

Another authority, Dr. Baldwin Tom, associate professor of immunology at the University of Texas Health Science Center, has revealed that, "AIDS researchers are keenly interested in natural substances like herbs that enhance the immune response." Dr. Tom said, "We have already identified plants that have an effect and there is good reason to investigate further."

In sufficient quantity, certain nutrients can "repair, rebuild and renew a tired immune system," according to Dr. Stuart Berger, developer of the Immune Power Diet. Dr. Berger says Vitamins B, C and E all play an important role in enhancing the immune system, along with calcium, magnesium, iron and zinc. Additional help comes from Vitamins A and D.

The best news of all comes from Dr. Paul Lee. Dr. Lee says, *"Taking certain herbs is the perfect health measure to protect yourself against AIDS."* Dr. Lee is a former director of the Academy of Herbal Studies in Santa Cruz, California and is a recognized authority on herbs.

Dr. Lee continues, "It would be of great value in treating diseases like AIDS and cancer to discover what ingredients in herbs stimulate the immune system and how to control them. The proper dose and combination of immune system-enhancing herbs can also be useful in treating AIDS patients.

"These herbs contain many active ingredients that stimulate the immune response, so taking them regularly will lower your risk, boost your health and prevent AIDS."

Dr. Lee points out, "Herbs are full of nutrients our food too often lacks, but which our immune system needs."

According to the experts, the following herbs are reputed to effectively enrich the body's immunological response and could therefore be considered as effective preventives against AIDS:

ECHINACEA (Echinacea augustifolia) - This plant is called Black Sampson (or Samson), Coneflower and Red Sunflower. The herb is currently under intensive investigation as an AIDS preventive. According to published herbals, Echinacea stimulates the production of white blood cells (leucocytes) and activates the vital enzyme *hyaluromidase,* thereby increasing the body's ability to resist infection. This herb contains essential oils, resins, and *echinoside,* an important blood cell normalizer. Echinacea is said to be a superior stimulant of the immune system and boosts the body's immunological response.

Echinacea is nontoxic and considered to be one of the most potent of the cleansing and purifying herbs. It improves the lymphatic system and assists lymphatic filtration and drainage and also helps remove toxins from the blood stream. Echinacea acts as a natural antibiotic and assists in removing bacteria, germs, and carcinogenic (cancer-causing) substances from the body.

Echinacea also contains the Vitamins A, C and E, along with iron, iodine, copper, sulphur and vital potassium. It is the root (rhizome) of this herb which provides its medicinal properties. Echinacea is a mild analgesic and a possible aphrodisiac. It has been used for centuries as a gargle, a compress for dental abcesses, and supplies the active ingredient for a healing salve. Dried and powdered Echinacea root may be purchased in most health food stores.

YERBAMATE (Ilex paraguariensis) - Although we know this herb as Yerbamate, the term comes to us from South America and is not actually the name of a plant, although it has come to be used as such. Yerbamate is an Americanized version of *Yerba* (herb) and *mate* (a tea-like beverage), pronounced 'mah-tay.'

Yerba Mate is widely cultivated in South America and is considered the national drink in both Paraguay and Brazil. It is estimated that the inhabitants of the South American continent consume more than 8 million pounds of Yerba Mate every year.

Yerba Mate is a tonic for the entire nervous system, is said to increase the body's resistance to disease, and to banish fatigue. It contains caffeine, but not in as strong a concentration as coffee. Yerba Mate also contains tannin, as do most commercial tea blends (except herbals), but is not as acid as either tea or coffee, making it much easier on the digestive tract.

However, more importantly, Yerba Mate is rich in iron, most trace minerals and Vitamins B, C and E, precisely the nutrients currently considered vital to the immune system. Yerba Mate is another natural preventive against AIDS because of its value in stimulating the body's all-important immunological response.

TAHEEBO/TECOMA (Bignoniaceae) - Taheebo, variously sold as *Tecoma, Tebebuia, Lapacho Colorado, Ipe Roxo* and *Pau D'Arco*, appears to be derived from the inner bark (cambrium) of one or more of the Tebebuia and/or Tecoma species trees. In South America, Taheebo is being investigated as a cure for cancer and other killer diseases. At the present time, American herbalists routinely use it against fungal and yeast infections. Taheebo is rich in iron, needed for efficient assimilation of nutrients and the elimination of the toxic waste byproducts of the body.

Taheebo is known as a potent natural antibiotic and is believed to contain elements the body needs to energize a tired immune system as well. The experts say Taheebo possesses antiviral properties, making it a powerful weapon against viral infestations like AIDS.

Note: In tracking down this elusive herbal, I discovered that Taheebo is actually an Indian tribal name for this medicinal and not a botanical designation. The name Ipe Roxo comes from Ipe, a small town near Bahia, Brazil, and roxo, meaning 'red.' The name Lapacho Colorado is Hispanic in origin and means 'red Lapacho,' and should not be confused with Lapacho morado, or 'purple Lapacho.' Pau D'Arco appears to be a corruption of a local name for one variety of Tecoma called Palo d'arco, meaning 'bow-wood.'

In doing the research for this chapter, I had a great deal of difficulty in finding authoritative, definitive information on this particular herbal. Many discrepancies exist. For instance, one piece of misinformation which seems to have been passed from writer to writer via the popular press is the statement that Tecoma/Tebebuia trees are insectivores, meaning that they feed on insects in much the same manner as the Venus Flytrap. Shame on these authors for not doing their homework and thereby perpetuating an error.

This information, while fascinating and sensational, is simply not true. Both Tecoma and Tebebuia put forth big, showy, trumpet-shaped flowers in many different brilliant hues, depending on the particular species. These flowers are very attractive to a number of different insects. The insects crawl into the heart of the flower to feast on the sweet nectar, become trapped, and are unable to extricate themselves. The flower does not close around the insect and assimilate it. If you peek into one of these blossoms, you will undoubtedly notice a plethora of insects trapped in its heart. This fact is certainly the source of the misconception.

ASTRALAGUS & LIGUSTRUM - Although they are not well-known in the U.S., both Astralagus and Ligustrum are in common use in China. That ancient land is considered the birthplace of the art of herbology and Chinese physicians are renowned around the world as skilled herbalists of the highest order.

Dr. Giora Mavligit of the University of Texas M.D. Anderson Hospital in Houston explained that these two herbs are used in China to boost the immune system and to battle cancer. Dr. Mavligit confirms that U.S. scientists and researchers have both Astralagus and Ligustrum under study at the present time.

In California, a company spokesman for Newport Pharmaceuticals in Newport Beach recently revealed that the immune-stimulating agents in these two herbs are under close laboratory study.

Note: Astralagus is sometimes known as Milk Vetch. Certain varieties of the 30 plants belonging to this species are known to be harmless. Some, like Loco Weed (A. wootonii), are poisonous and cause loco disease in cattle and other pasture animals who find it tasty.

Ligustrum belongs to the privet family, of which there are more than 50 varieties. In fact, you or a neighbor may have a handsome privet hedge. Certain dense privets are often clipped into animal shapes or fanciful figures. Privet is commonly used for skillfully clipped topiary sculptures.

The plant contains tannin, resins, mannitol (a sweetish carbohydrate), and ligustrin (a form of detergent). Ligustrum is used in herbal medicine externally as a healing and cleansing agent for open wounds. Like Mistletoe, its berries are very poisonous. Authoritative texts caution that internal use should be avoided. Ligustrum is said to produce severe abdominal symptoms.

As you can see from the above, the use of Astralagus and Ligustrum should be left to the discretion of informed health professionals. We cannot recommend either of these two powerful herbs for self-administration. Until ongoing research establishes a safe recommended dosage or safe method of preparation, it appears best to adopt a 'wait and see' attitude.

HOW IS THE AIDS VIRUS TRANSMITTED TO OTHERS? - All over America, parents are taking their children out of school when a classmate is known to have AIDS. Schools are being picketed and children infected with AIDS are being reviled and ostracized, sometimes by school personnel as well as by parents and classmates.

Before they will agree to perform, certain actresses are demanding to know whether their male co-stars have AIDS. Homosexual actors are being shunned and love scenes are being written out of scripts.

Nurses and even doctors in some hospitals and health-care facilities are refusing to work with patients who have AIDS. Authorities are forced to admit that AIDS has reached epidemic proportions in the United States.

As a nation, are we overreacting to the threat posed by this killer virus? Science says AIDS is not as easily contracted as most people think. Just exactly how safe are we? What do we need to guard against, and what contact with an AIDS victim carries a risk? Should children with AIDS be allowed to attend school and associate with healthy children?

Dr. Anthony Fauci, director of the National Institute of Allergy & Infectious Diseases in Bethesda, Maryland, and Dr. Martha Rogers, a specialist with the AIDS branch of the Federal Center for Disease Control in Atlanta, Georgia, were closely questioned recently. Their answers were reassuring.

The Center for Disease Control has stated that there are no identified cases of AIDS in the U.S. known to have been transmitted in schools, day-care centers or foster-care facilities, or even through casual person-to-person contact. "Mandatory screening for AIDS as a condition for entry of schools is not warranted," says the CDC.

The AIDS task force of the U.S. Department of Public Health has determined that most children with AIDS should be allowed to attend school, but recommends that certain children with the disease be placed in special circumstances. Children who have neurological handicaps, those with oozing sores, and those who have no control over their bowels or bladder will be isolated from the healthy children.

As of late 1985, there were 164 children under the age of thirteen in the United States who suffer from AIDS. Studies show that the vast majority of these unfortunate victims got the disease from the blood of their infected mothers, either during pregnancy or at birth.

Dr. Dean Echenberg, chief of communicable disease control at the State Department of Public Health in San Francisco, says, "Studies of children of parents with AIDS have shown there is no family-to-child transmission or child-to-child transmission of the disease." According to Dr. Echenberg, these studies show the risk of developing AIDS by living with (or visiting) an infected person is almost nonexistent.

Research shows that the AIDS virus cannot pass through skin, but must enter the body through the mouth, other orifices, mucous membranes or open wounds. Authorities say the virus cannot long survive outside the body.

As most people are aware, AIDS is contracted mainly through sexual intercourse, although an infected hypodermic needle or transfusion of blood containing the virus will transmit it quite readily to a healthy person. However, authorities say large quantities of AIDS-infected body fluids (blood, semen or sexual discharges) must directly enter the body. (Note: All donated blood is now routinely screened for AIDS. The CDC says blood transfusions are completely safe.)

The AIDS virus has not been found in perspiration, urine or feces. It is true that very low levels of the virus have been identified in tears and saliva, but researchers say a much higher concentration would have to be present before even deep kissing (where saliva intermingles) represents a real risk, unless there are open sores in the mouth or on the lips. Kissing, coughing, sneezing and spitting is unlikely to spread the disease.

(Note: Because it is at least *theoretically* possible that AIDS might be transmitted through saliva, although the risk is minimal, Federal officials have recommended keeping AIDS-infected children who have a tendency to bite or scratch out of the classroom.)

Authorities say there is no evidence that the AIDS virus can be caught from toilet seats, showers or objects in common use in the home, school or locker room. In addition, there is no evidence that eating food prepared by an infected person, either at home or in a restaurant, is a risk. And, because chlorine kills the virus, AIDS cannot be contracted by sharing a swimming pool with an infected person.

The Department of Public Health has pointed out that over ten thousand doctors, nurses, technicians and specialists have taken care of AIDS patients since this killer was first recognized. In the course of their duties, health-care personnel have been exposed to the virus for long periods of time. Family members who care for an AIDS victim at home have also been exposed for long periods.

As in all communicable diseases, routine precautions should be taken when caring for an infected person. According to the authorities, efficient disinfecting procedures should be practiced when cleaning patients and handling their body fluids. However, it should be emphasized that the only known case of a health-care worker contracting the virus was that of a nurse in Britain who developed AIDS after accidentally infecting herself with an AIDS-contaminated needle.

IS THERE A FINAL SOLUTION? - All over the country, researchers are working overtime attempting to find the final solution to AIDS. Certainly science will eventually develop a vaccine against this killer disease or find a way to reactivate and restore a damaged and disintegrating immune system.

In the meantime, let us hope that the hysteria provoked by the very thought of AIDS will be replaced by sober, thoughtful action. Above all, be sure your sexual partner is clean and healthy. Don't over-react if you find a friend, neighbor or classmate of your child has AIDS. If you find yourself unavoidably in contact with an AIDS victim, follow the same precautions you would with any communicable disease. Remember the miracle cure-all herbs that are to be found in Nature's Pharmacy and take them regularly to provide your immune system with the ammunition it needs to continue to function fully and normally.

Chapter 38
COMMON PROBLEMS & THEIR HERBAL HELPERS

INTRODUCTION: As you have undoubtedly noticed in the previous chapters, combinations of herbs often complement one another and, in some instances, the combination proves more efficacious than a single herb used by itself.

Although you will find herbs used in these combinations that may not be mentioned elsewhere in this book, this is only because space would not allow a chapter on every medicinal plant found in Nature's Pharmacy. The herbs selected for in-depth presentation in the chapter material are the most universally acknowledged for their medicinal properties, but there are others equally as effective, and still more which potentiate the whole when used in a blend. If you wish, you may refer to the individual chapters on selected medicinals (where applicable) for additional information.

Note: In many instances, you will find a large quantity of a certain infusion is recommended. When taken in small sips every fifteen minutes or so throughout the waking hours, the entire daily allotment can be easily tolerated.

HOW TO PREPARE: The most popular method of ingesting herbs is in an infusion, or tea. Unless otherwise indicated, you may use any of the medicinal plants listed below singly or as a blend.

When preparing combination teas, simply mix equal amounts (or quantities specified) of the fresh or dried herbs together and use one heaping teaspoon of the blend for every 6 ounces of freshly boiled water. Steep, covered, for three to five minutes (depending on the strength you prefer), strain and add honey to taste.

This next direction is very important: Kick off your shoes, put your feet up, slip a pillow under your head, lean back and sip hot. Sure, you can grab a cup standing at the kitchen counter, but do yourself a favor and take twenty minutes to relax and let the healing qualities of the appropriate herbal blend warm and soothe your entire body.

ACNE: A useful treatment for acne traditionally includes sipping up to one quart daily of kidney-cleansing Stinging Nettle tea. Because disfiguring pimples are often caused by sluggish kidneys, this internal cleansing should be assisted by adhering to a diet from which chocolate, fats, strongly spiced, excessively salty and acid foods are removed in order to give the kidneys the rest they need.

The external application of horseradish vinegar greatly potentiates the entire treatment. Prepare the vinegar by coarsely shredding a small quantity of horseradish into a glass (not plastic) bottle. Add a mild wine or fruit vinegar to cover and allow the blend to stand at room temperature for a few days. Smooth the liquid on a wet face mornings and evenings and allow it to remain for ten minutes before rinsing off with cool water. You will be surprised to find that this blend produces a mild tincture which dries and heals even pustulant eruptions without the heat of the horseradish or the sharpness of the vinegar.

AMPUTATED LIMBS: Many times one of the most agonizing problems an amputee must face is a lingering pain that appears to be based in the portion of the limb which has been removed. A 'ghost pain' of this type is often relieved by the application of Comfrey poultices. Continuing applications have been known to conquer the sensation entirely.

Another treatment which may bring relief from ghost pain is rubbing an onion tincture on the stump. The tincture is easily prepared by filling a glass bottle with thinly sliced onion. Add pure spirits to cover and allow the tincture to stand in a warm place for ten days. Strain and bottle the resulting essence and apply as often as necessary, rubbing in well.

Bathing the stump with an infusion of Thyme thrice weekly can also ease ghost pain. Prepare the infusion with a heaping handful of dried or fresh Thyme. This infusion may be rewarmed and used three times in all. Sleeping with a Thyme and Club Moss pillow cushioning the stump will help relieve ghost pain as well.

Internally, an infusion (tea) made from the thoroughly dried and ground roots of the Iris assists in eliminating ghost pain also. A coffee or seed grinder makes the grinding easy. Soak one-half teaspoonful of the powdered root in 6 ounces of cold water overnight and sip one to two cups throughout the day.

APPENDIX (IRRITATED): "Taking a cup of Blackberry leaf tea soothes an irritated appendix almost immediately," says a traditional European folk healer. Some herbologists believe the action of the Blackberry leaf is so powerful that a possible attack of appendicitis might be avoided by the regular use of this infusion.

APPETITE (POOR): A child with no appetite or a convalescent patient will regain their appetites by sipping Stinging Nettle tea. A complement to this treatment is the use of a full Thyme bath. Rosy cheeks and a healthy hunger soon follow.

ARTHRITIS: See Joints

BLADDER: Burning, painful urination is a symptom of cystitis, an inflammation or infection of the bladder most often afflicting women. Cystitis causes lower back pain and the patient may run a fever. Other afflictions of the bladder include bed-wetting and the abnormal retention of urine, which calls for a diuretic.

The particular herbs traditionally used in bladder complaints include: Lady's Mantle (cleansing), Chamomile (a gastro-intestinal tonic), Parsley (stimulates copious urine), Dandelion (neutralizes acid), Uva Ursi (tonic for urinary tract), and Juniper Berries (assists in clearing infection). Either Yarrow or Horsetail may be used in a sitz bath and both are noted for bringing quick relief.

BLOOD: The toxins and impurities which build up in the blood may be carried to the vital organs by the blood stream, thus weakening the entire body. Faulty nutrition, environmental pollution and various illnesses can all contribute to 'bad' blood.

The cleansing, purifying herbs include: Dandelion Root (cleanser and detoxifier), Burdock (aids kidney function), Yarrow (blood purifier), Barberry (stimulates bile flow), Red Clover (tonic).

BONES (WEAK): At least one authority on herbs recommends the use of the ground seeds of Fenugreek to build and strengthen weak bones caused by osteoporosis, osteomyelitis and certain conditions manifested by an atrophy of the bone itself. The recommended method is to add one-half teaspoon of ground Fenugreek seeds to a half cup of Yarrow tea. Take two half-cups thus prepared and two half-cups of plain Yarrow tea daily.

Prepare a Yarrow bath using two double handfuls of the herb and soak for twenty minutes (with the chest region out of the water) once a month. The bath may be used three times in all. It is said that a tincture of Yarrow smoothed into the body greatly assists this bone strengthening treatment.

BONES/TEETH: A lack of calcium, or the inability to assimilate calcium, leads to brittle bones, tooth decay, bleeding gums, insomnia, lower back pain and muscle cramps. Not surprisingly, nature has provided herbs rich in easily assimilated calcium.

The bone building herbs include: Comfrey (contains calcium and phosphorus), Irish Moss (high in calcium), Horsetail (calcium and silica), Oat Straw (calcium, phosphorus, silica), Hops (as a potentiating agent). (Note: Please also see MOUTH this chapter.)

BOWELS: Sluggish bowels and chronic constipation can allow toxic wastes to enter the bloodstream and travel through the body. Overuse of harsh chemical laxatives may result in a complete loss of normal functioning of the entire intestinal tract.

The natural aids for normal bowel function include: Stinging Nettle (stimulates peristalsis), Yarrow (regulates movements), Barberry (promotes bile), Licorice (mildly laxative), Mallow (soothes inflammation), Capsicum (stimulant and purifier). Note: Taking one tablespoon of cold-processed, unrefined linseed oil daily with a little liquid improves digestion and will normalize bowel dysfunction.

BREATH (BAD): A person suffering from chronic halitosis (bad breath) needs the advice of a physician to determine the cause of the condition. Common causes of bad breath include decaying teeth, canker sores or ulcerated membranes of the mouth, tonsillitis, post-nasal drip, low levels of stomach acid resulting in poor digestion, or even long-term constipation.

A visit to your dentist will take care of bad teeth. Try rinsing with a warm infusion of Cleavers for canker sores or ulcers of the mouth and use a deep gargle of Sage tea to soothe inflammed tonsils. Sniffing warm Sage tea will aid in clearing the nasal passages and helps clear up even a bad case of post-nasal drip.

Sipping a few drops of Juniper oil diluted in a glass of water or chewing a few dill seeds freshens the breath quickly. Regular gargling with thirty to forty drops of Myrrh tincture mixed in a glass of lukewarm water helps eliminate bad breath when it is caused by a disorder of the oral cavity.

BREATHING (LABORED): Conditions which cause labored breathing and shortness of breath include emphysema, cardiac asthma and a dysfunction of the thyroid gland. Many herbalists believe the root of the problem lies in a disorder of the liver which results in pressure and swelling of the bronchial tubes. For this condition, take one cup of Club Moss tea every morning upon arising and apply a Swedish Bitters compress to the liver for four hours during the day. A Horsetail poultice applied overnight to the region of the liver greatly strengthens the treatment.

CATARACTS/GLAUCOMA: Many holistic herbalists believe glaucoma is complicated by a kidney dysfunction and may often be accompanied by rheumatic pain. A tea made from equal parts of Stinging Nettle, Speedwell, Calendula and Horsetail with one teaspoon of Swedish Bitters added should be taken daily. A Horsetail sitz bath aids in potentiating the treatment.

Swedish Bitters brushed across the eyelids is said to be an effective treatment for cataracts. In addition, a cotton pad moistened with Swedish Bitters can be laid across the closed eyes to relieve pain.

A steam bath for the eyes reputed to clear dim vision is made as follows: Blend together 20 grams Eyebright, 20 grams Valerian, 10 grams Vervain, 30 grams Elder Flowers and 20 grams Chamomile. Bring one pint of white wine to boiling and pour over 5 level tablespoons of the blended herbs. Drape a towel over your head, close your eyes and allow the fragrant steam to bathe and penetrate the closed eyelids.

Note: Please see EYES this chapter for additional tips for bright, healthy eyes.

COLON: Complaints of the colon may present themselves in the form of abdominal pain, diarrhea, constipation, indigestion or as a serious inflammation which results in irritable colon, colitis or dysentery. A healthy colon processes and excretes waste efficiently and is vital to a healthy body.

The herbs thought most beneficial to a healthy colon include: Calamus (strengthens and stimulates), Calendula (reduces inflammation), Comfrey (heals and strengthens), Mallow (coats and soothes irritation), Hops (relaxes).

CONSTIPATION: One of the healthiest ways to conquer constipation forever is to take 3 tablespoons of linseed oil with a little liquid each meal. The healthy polyunsaturated fats in pure, cold-processed, unrefined linseed oil will normalize the entire digestive tract.

You probably already know that prunes effectively relieve constipation, but did you know that figs work equally well? *Fig Rolls* are an old European folk remedy and are easily made. Mince 1 pound of fresh figs and add 1 ounce of finely ground Senna leaves. Form the mass into rolls, wrap tightly in aluminum foil, and store refrigerated. Every morning before breakfast, take a piece the size of the tip of your little finger until movements have become normal.

An infusion of Wild Chicory will stimulate the bowels almost immediately. One cup of this tea is most beneficial taken on an empty stomach upon arising in the morning. Don't be surprised if you find you have a bowel movement after each meal. And don't worry either. Nature designed our bodies to evacuate everytime we eat, but modern over-processed foods often do not provide the necessary stimulation.

DIABETES: Although they cannot take the place of prescribed medicines, certain herbal remedies have been shown to aid in disorders of the pancreas, including diabetes and hypoglycemia. Please see PANCREAS this chapter.

EYES: There is no better remedy for visual problems caused by a Vitamin A deficiency than the common carrot (see Chapter 6). If you have a problem with your eyes, please try carrot juice.

The herbs said to aid in strengthening weak, strained and irritated eyes include: Eyebright (builds immunity to infection), Golden Seal (natural antibiotic), Bayberry (aids eye membranes), Yarrow (relieves congestion).

FATIGUE: If you lack energy and awaken tired in the morning, a visit to the doctor is certainly indicated to determine the root cause.

However, a thyroid problem resulting in a sluggish metabolism is one common cause of chronic fatigue, as are too little exercise and too much food.

Several herbs act to stimulate the system, including: Calamus (cleanser and tonic), Mistletoe (aids hormonal secretions), Capsicum (assists circulation), Gotu Kola (stimulates and strengthens), Ginseng (powers the brain).

FEMALE COMPLAINTS: The wide range of female complaints include PMS (premenstrual syndrome), menstrual cramps, irregular menstruation and the characteristic discomforts of menopause, such as hot flashes and irritability.

The 'women's herbs' include: Lady's Mantle (astringent and healing), Red Raspberry Leaves (tones uterine muscles), Black Cohosh (natural hormonal action), Mallow (soothes mucous membranes), Yarrow (lessens spasms and normalizes female organs).

An excellent combination tea which can normalize excessive menstrual flow can be made from two parts Valerian and one part each Arnica, Balm Mint, Iceland Moss, Sage and Yarrow. Blend well and use one heaping teaspoon for every 6 ounces of freshly boiled water. Cover and steep for three minutes. Regular use of this infusion is reputed to correct abnormal menstrual flow and to insure a smooth passage through menopause with no unpleasant symptoms.

Those unfortunate women who cannot seem to carry a baby full-term and who miscarry often may be assisted by taking Lady's Mantle and Yarrow regularly. Additional help can be found by boiling three leaves of young Hornbeam shoots in milk. Beat in the yolk of an egg and add a rich white sauce to create a healthy soup. Take the soup as dinner regularly for good nutrition.

GALL BLADDER: Nature's Pharmacy may provide relief from the nausea, vomiting and pain caused by gall stones. It is said that a six-week treatment with the extracted juice of the black radish can, in some cases, dissolve small stones. Begin by extracting 3 ounces and increase intake gradually to 12 ounces by the third week. Over the last three weeks of treatment, decrease intake gradually back to 3 ounces. Note: Black radish juice is acid and should not be taken if the intestines or stomach are irritated or inflamed.

Another herbal treatment for gall stones consists of blending equal amounts of Agrimony, Hops, Lesser Burnet, Peppermint and Wormwood. Put three tablespoons of the blended herbs into a quart of apple wine and bring just to the boiling point. Steep for three minutes and strain into a thermos to keep hot. Take one tablespoon of the hot liquid every waking hour during the day.

GLANDULARS: Glandular secretions regulate many of the vital functions of the body. To keep the glands healthy, certain nutrients are required.

The following medicinals are reputed to stimulate glandular-hormonal secretions: Mistletoe (aids glandular secretions), Dandelion Root (stimulates and strengthens glands), Alfalfa (increases secretions and nourishes system), Kelp (natural iodine stimulates and reactivates glands).

HEADACHES: Headache pain may range from a dull ache to an annoying throbbing to the acute almost unbearable pain of a migraine. Headaches may be caused by congested (or infected) sinuses, a high fever, a stomach or digestive disorder, or even breathing polluted air. Headaches can be triggered by something as simple as emotional stress or something as serious as a brain tumor.

The pain-relieving herbs include: Horsetail (reduces inflammation), Comfrey (internal cleanser), Alfalfa (contains alkaloids), Yucca (similar to cortisone), Burdock (reduces swelling), Valerian (relaxant).

HEALERS: The following combination of herbs aids in healing 'breaks' in the body, including broken bones (fractures) and even open wounds of all kinds. The prime ingredient, Comfrey, is often called 'Knitbone.'

The healing herbs include: Comfrey (stimulates healing), Golden Seal (natural antibiotic), Mallow (soothes inflammations), Shepherd's Purse (aids clotting).

HEART: One of the primary causes of heart disease is arteriosclerosis, better known as hardening of the arteries. In this condition, the blood vessels which feed the heart become clogged with plaque. The first overt sign of the disease may be a disabling or even fatal heart attack.

The cleansing and strengthening herbs for the heart traditionally include: Horsetail (diuretic and blood purifier), Hawthorne (organic cardiac tonic), Garlic (strengthens vessels and overcomes infections), Capsicum (potentiates).

A superior and pleasant tea said to aid in heart problems by helping to restore normal circulation consists of blending three parts Hawthorne, two parts each Mistletoe and Yerba Mate with one part each Arnica, Balm Mint, Bean Pods, Bladder Wrack, Burdock, Burnet (Lesser), Calamus, Couch Grass, Dandelion, Frangula Bark, Fumitory, Horsetail, Irish Moss, Knotgrass, Motherwort, Nettle (Hemp), Rue, Shepherd's Purse, Silverweed, Rest-Harrow, and Yarrow.

Because some of these delicate herbs cannot tolerate heat, use one heaping teaspoon of the blend for every 6 ounces of cold water and steep overnight. The following morning, heat slightly for palatability, sweeten with a teaspoon of honey, and take one cup mornings and one cup evenings.

HICCOUGHS: When all else fails, try a teaspoon of Dill Seeds steeped for three minutes in 6 ounces of freshly boiled water. Do not sweeten this soothing remedy. Sip hot and the involuntary spasms of the most stubborn hiccoughs will be relieved.

HYPERTENSION (HIGH BLOOD PRESSURE): High blood pressure is often called the 'silent killer' because the condition causes no pain until it explodes in a stroke or heart attack. All adults should have their blood pressure monitored regularly.

Note: If you are on medication, *do not* stop taking your medicine. Herbs can be a useful adjunct to your prescription, and may act to prevent the condition from occurring in the first place, but only your doctor can change or discontinue your medication.

The natural medicinals which aid in normalizing blood pressure include: Garlic (purifies and helps stabilize), Capsicum (stimulates and potentiates), Shepherd's Purse (normalizes), Golden Seal (natural antibiotic), Parsley (mild diuretic).

HYPOGLYCEMIA: This condition, caused by an imbalance in the system resulting in abnormally low blood sugar, can only be diagnosed by a glucose tolerance test administered by a physician, and is becoming more and more common. Symptoms include chronic fatigue, mood swings, restlessness, irritability and a marked weakness. To a large degree, hypoglycemia and hyperglycemia can be conquered by a change in diet.

Helps from the plant kingdom include: Dandelion Root (helps balance blood), Safflower (stimulates adrenals and pancreas), Garlic (natural antibiotic and cleanser), Licorice Root (quick energy).

INFECTIONS: Any bacterial or viral infection in the body results in inflammation, swollen glands and soreness and may be accompanied by a fever. Forcing liquids and stimulating copious perspiration assists the immune system in its battle against infections of all kinds.

Herbal helps include: Golden Seal (natural antibiotic), Plantain (neutralizes poisons), Mallow (healing and soothing), Yarrow (blood cleanser), Echinacea (gland cleanser).

INFLUENZA (FLU): Because the various types of flu are caused by a virus, they are difficult to treat medically. Common symptoms include alternating chills and fever, vomiting and diarrhea, a sore throat and headaches.

The following combination of soothing herbs can help make a bout of the flu more bearable: Golden Seal (natural antibiotic), Mallow (to coat and quiet inflammation), Licorice (relieves coughs), Capsicum (stimulates, reduces fever, potentiates), Ginseng (an energizer).

INSOMNIA: If you suffer from occasional bouts of sleeplessness caused by stress, anxiety or worry, don't worry. Help is at hand.

Avoid caffeine drinks, of course, and leisurely sip a cup of honeyed Cowslip (or Valerian) tea before retiring brewed with one heaping teaspoon of the herb of your choice for every 6 ounces of freshly boiled water. Steep for three minutes.

JOINTS: Joint pain, often accompanied by swelling, stiffness and inflammation, is a common symptom of arthritis, rheumatism, neuritis and bursitis. The pain-relieving herbs include: Horsetail (reduces inflammation), Comfrey (internal cleanser), Alfalfa (contains alkaloids), Yucca (similar to cortisone), Burdock (reduces swelling), Valerian (relaxant).

The holistic treatment favored in Europe recommends taking one cup of Horsetail tea one-half hour before breakfast and another cup one-half hour before the last meal of the day. The regimen suggests adding one tablespoon of Swedish Bitters to one-half cup of Stinging Nettle tea. Sip a portion before each of the three daily meals and the remainder after the meal. A total of four cups of Stinging Nettle should be taken during the waking hours.

A Horsetail poultice may be left in place overnight and can often relieve stiffness. In addition, a brisk massage with a tincture of Comfrey is reputed to reduce swelling. Another overnight treatment recommended abroad is the application of Cow-Parsnip leaves, Hogweed or cabbage leaves (warmed with an iron). A twenty-minute Horsetail sitz bath of the affected area is said to be very beneficial as well.

KIDNEYS: The kidneys are part of the all-important waste removal system of the body and assist in maintaining the electrolyte and acid content of the blood. Healthy kidneys are vital to a healthy body.

Herbal aids for healthy kidneys include: Golden Rod (astringent and diuretic), Dead Nettle (blood purifier), Cleavers (diuretic and tonic), Mallow (soothes irritation), Uva Ursi (solvent).

Authoritative herbals recommend a tea made from equal parts of Agrimony, Birch Leaves, Rest-Harrow and Shepherd's Purse to aid in dissolving and expelling stones and gravel in the gall bladder as well as the kidneys. Horsetail tea and sitz baths greatly aid in potentiating the treatment.

LIVER: The liver is the largest organ of the body and performs many important functions. It absorbs, filters, detoxifies, excretes and stores certain elements necessary to life maintenance. Liver complaints include cirrhosis, hepatitis and cancer.

The herbs thought beneficial to liver function include: Greater Celandine (diuretic and mild purgative), Dandelion Root (stimulant and detoxifier), Chamomile (healer and purifier), Golden Rod (stimulates healing), Horsetail (builds and tones), Parsley (cleanses and nourishes). (Note: See LIVER, Chapter 39, for additional information.)

LUNGS: Inflammation or infection of the lungs may be caused by croup, bronchitis, smoking or even air pollution. All increase mucous congestion, which in turn triggers coughing.

Herbal helpers for lung congestion include: Plantain (cleanses), Comfrey (dissolves mucous), Stinging Nettle (clears congestion), Mallow (soothes irritation), Mullein (natural antibiotic). (Note: See LUNGS, Chapter 39, for additional information.)

MOUTH: For receeding gums, gingivitis and loose teeth, a blending of equal amounts of Knotgrass, Lady's Mantle, Oak Bark and Sage should be prepared as a cold infusion overnight using two heaping teaspoons of the blend for every 8 ounces of cold water. Warm slightly and store in a thermos to maintain temperature. Swish the infusion around the mouth repeatedly during the day and use a toothbrush dipped in the tea to massage the gums. (Note: See BONES/TEETH this chapter for additional information.)

MUSCLE DISORDERS: Nature's Pharmacy provides some potent herbal helpers which are reputed to work slowly but surely against muscle disorders, including *multiple sclerosis.* The same herbs are said to aid certain handicapped and spastic children, those who suffer from speech disorders, and those born with Down's Syndrome (Mongoloid).

The affected muscles should be massaged briskly thrice daily with a tincture of Shepherd's Purse. Other tinctures which aid these conditions when used in a massage include Comfrey, St. John's Wort, Chamomile and Yarrow. Lady's Mantle tea and Sage tea should be sipped throughout the day.

Comforting sitz baths concocted from Chamomile, Horsetail, Pine sprigs, Sage, St. John's Wort, Thyme or Yarrow are suggested. A Thyme or Stinging Nettle bath stimulates circulation. These herbs are noted for having a beneficial effect on weak muscles.

PALSY: (Parkinson's Disease) may yield to the extracted juice of the Wood Sorrel. The recommended method is to dilute three to five drops of Wood Sorrel juice in a cup of Yarrow tea made with 1 heaping teaspoon of Yarrow for every 6 ounces of freshly boiled water. Ingest up to five cups daily. Apply a Swedish Bitters compress to the back of the head for a period of four hours and briskly massage the spine with a tincture of Yarrow. Thyme baths relieve sore and stiff muscles as well.

Sitz baths or full baths made with Pine Sprigs, St. John's Wort, Chamomile, Sage, Stinging Nettle, Yarrow, Thyme and Horsetail are reputed to assist in overcoming paralysis and atrophy. (See General Directions, Chapter 2, for how to prepare.) The patient should relax in the bath for twenty minutes and then spend a full hour warmly covered in bed and perspiring. Use only one herb for each bath and vary the herbs used daily to stimulate circulation.

A soothing whole-body poultice of Cow-Parsnip leaves left on overnight often brings amazing results. Crush the leaves well with a wooden rolling pin and spread out on a sheet. Wrap the patient in the sheet and cover warmly. This poultice may remain in place overnight unless the patient complains of discomfort in sensitive areas. If discomfort occurs, the patient must be unwrapped immediately. Most report a feeling of comforting warmth and sleep deeply and well.

NERVOUS COMPLAINTS: A nervous disorder can be caused by improper nutrition, overwork, anxiety, noise-pollution and both physical and emotional problems. An overstimulated, highly excitable individual is strongly affected by stress and emotions and is often characterized as 'nervous.'

The relaxing nerve-soothing herbals include: Valerian (reduces tension), Speedwell (dispels depression), Mistletoe (nature's tranquilizer), Hops (nature's sedative), Black Cohosh (nourishes weak nerves), St. John's Wort (pain reliever).

PANCREAS: The pancreatic gland produces insulin, which regulates blood sugar levels in the blood, and aids digestion with pancreatic enzymes. Diabetes is caused by a dysfunction of the pancreas.

The pancreatic stimulating herbs include: Calamus, Dandelion, Mistletoe and Stinging Nettle. (Note: Please see appropriate chapters for instruction on preparation.)

A special infusion which may benefit the diabetic is prepared as follows: Blend together 3 tablespoons each Avens (Geum alpina) and Golden Fingergrass (Potentilla auria), 2 tablespoons dried green bean pods and 1 tablespoon each Blackberry leaves and Blueberry leaves. Use 1 level teaspoon of the blended herbs for every 6 ounces of freshly boiled water. Steep, covered, for three minutes. Up to two quarts daily of this infusion may be taken.

PROSTATE: It has been reliably stated that every male over the age of fifty will suffer some involvement of the prostate with increasing age. The most common condition, prostatitis, is an inflammation of the gland.

In the entire pharmacopeia of herbal medicine, the Willow Herb (see Chapter 33) is by far the greatest aid in any involvement of the prostate. Additional natural aids for a healthy prostate include: Golden Seal (reduces inflammation), Parsley (fights infection), Mallow (nourishes tissues), Juniper Berries (antiseptic properties), Capsicum (stimulates and reduces swellings).

RESPIRATORY COMPLAINTS: The list of common respiratory complaints includes colds, coughs, bronchitis, allergies, hay fever and asthma.

The herbs found effective against these conditions include: Stinging Nettle (soothes inflammation), Golden Seal (natural antibiotic), Capsicum (strong stimulant), Parsley (tonic and cleanser), Mallow (coats and soothes mucous membranes).

Stinging Nettle is particularly beneficial in cases of allergic reaction, such as seasonal hay fever. Stir three teaspoons of Swedish Bitters into an infusion of Stinging Nettle and take up to four cups daily for quick relief.

When a severe cold or sinus infection acts to block the ears, a warm infusion of Ground Ivy, Sage and Yarrow is used as a rinse of the affected passages to help relieve the blockage which is making hearing difficult. Another folk remedy which is remarkably effective is placing a bit of cotton moistened with Swedish Bitters into the ear after first dropping warm Thyme oil into the passage to insure no irritation occurs from the alcohol in the Swedish Bitters.

SHINGLES: Anyone who has ever suffered the agonizing pain of Shingles will be interested to know that the juice of Leeks (Sempervivum tectorum) can bring quick relief. Cut the fleshy leaves and allow the juice to collect in a saucer or use a juice extractor. Smooth this fragrant juice on the affected parts.

SKIN: Did you know that the skin is the largest eliminative system of the body? When the skin is functioning properly, a great many toxins are excreted through normal perspiration. But the skin cannot do the job alone. Clear, healthy skin greatly depends on the efficient functioning of the blood, lymph, liver and kidneys. Strengthening the detoxifying and purifying systems of the body aids the skin as well.

The purifying herbs include: Cleavers (strengthens), Horsetail (internal tonic), Sage (astringent), Calamus (internal cleanser), Kelp (nourishes). Note: A good scrubbing with a rough washcloth or loofah when bathing stimulates, tones, removes dead cells from the surface of the skin and opens the pores thereby making it easier for the skin to do its work of excreting toxins.

Psoriasis and *eczema* are two skin conditions which may be aided by a herbal infusion consisting of five parts Stinging Nettle, four parts Goat's Beard, three parts each Willow Bark, Greater Celandine, Speedwell and Calendula, two parts each Fumitory, Walnut Husks and Yarrow and one part Oak Bark. After blending, use one heaping teaspoon for every 6 ounces of freshly boiled water and steep, covered, for three minutes. Sip up to two quarts of this tea daily.

The typical cracking, scaling and itching of affected parts can be relieved by using an ointment prepared with the extracted juice of the Greater Celandine combined with pure lard (not shortening). (See Chapter 2 for instructions on preparing an ointment.)

Baths of equal parts of Mallow and Horsetail act to coat, soothe and speed healing. The patient should relax in the bath for twenty minutes at a time with the chest out of the water. (See General Directions, Chapter 2, for preparing a bath.)

STROKE (PREVENTIVE MEASURES): Authoritative herbalists recommend an infusion of equal parts of Angelica, Avens, Five-Leaf Grass, Hyssop, Lavender, Marjoram, Masterwort, Rosemary, Sage, Silverweed, Sweet Violet and Valerian. Pour 6 ounces of apple cider heated to just boiling over one heaping teaspoon of the blend and steep for three minutes. It is said that this tea prepared and taken fresh several times daily may prevent a stroke even if mild symptoms (such as anxiety, dizziness, restlessness or a pull of the facial muscles) are present. However, any unusual symptoms are an immediate signal to consult your doctor.

A moderate diet and slow daily walks are beneficial. No tobacco, coffee and alcohol (except Swedish Bitters) should be taken. A cold infusion of Mistletoe can help if one cup is taken upon arising and another cup is taken before retiring. In addition to the Mistletoe regimen, two cups of Sage tea should be sipped during the day and a Swedish Bitters compress applied to the heart region.

STROKE (PARALYZING): After a paralyzing stroke, the patient may benefit from a traditional six-week Mistletoe treatment consisting of ingesting three cups of the infusion daily for a period of three weeks, two cups daily for a period of two weeks, and one cup daily for the final week. Because Mistletoe is prepared as a cold infusion, it is recommended that the daily allotment be heated to lukewarm in the morning and stored in a thermos to maintain a comfortable sipping temperature.

An alternate treatment consists of blending equal portions of Balm, Lavender, Rosemary, Sage, Speedwell and St. John's Wort. Use one heaping teaspoon of the mixed herbs for every 6 ounces of freshly boiled water. Take one cup in the morning and one cup in the afternoon daily.

Chapter 39

MALIGNANCIES & THEIR HERBAL HELPERS

Although the following medicinal plants are believed to be a useful adjunct to conventional medical treatment of various cancers, the reader is cautioned to seek competent medical advice at the first warning sign of any malignancy.

BLOOD (LEUKEMIA): A combination of various herbs is reputed to be successful against this insidious condition. Blend together three parts each Calendula, Elder Shoots, Greater Celandine and Stinging Nettle, two and one-half parts each Bedstraw, Goat's Beard and Yarrow, and one and one-half parts each Dandelion Roots and St. John's Wort. Use one heaping teaspoon of the mixed herbs for every 6 ounces of freshly boiled water. Cover and steep for three minutes. Sip up to two quarts of this infusion daily.

Because many herbalists believe the origin of leukemia is the spleen, six *sips* (not cups) of Calamus Root tea should be taken. (Note: Calamus is prepared as a cold infusion. See Chapter 4 for complete directions.) The recommended method is to take one sip before and one sip after each of the three main meals of the day. In addition, up to three tablespoons of Swedish Bitters daily should be taken under the following regimen: Stir one tablespoon of Swedish Bitters into a cup of herb tea. Sip one-half cup before and one-half cup after each of the three daily meals.

To further potentiate the treatment, a Swedish Bitters compress may be applied to the spleen and liver for four hours. A warm Horsetail poultice applied to the affected region overnight is also believed to be of benefit.

BONE: Yarrow is a powerful herb reputed to stimulate the production of healthy bone marrow. Up to four cups daily may be taken. To aid in purifying the blood, two cups of Calendula tea and two cups of Stinging Nettle tea should be sipped throughout the waking hours. Add one tablespoon of Swedish Bitters to one cup of the herbal brew and take one-half cup before and one-half cup after each of the three daily meals. Either Swedish Bitters or a tincture of Yarrow or Comfrey should be used in a brisk massage several times daily.

BREAST: After an operation to excise (remove) a tumor of the breast tissue, including a partial or complete mastectomy, Calendula ointment will assist in restoring skin tone and can prevent the pain of healing tissue. In addition, scarring may be minimized. A Swedish Bitters compress or Horsetail poultice can also relieve pain.

An infusion prepared with three parts Calendula and one part each Stinging Nettle and Yarrow should be taken. Use one heaping teaspoon of the blend for each 6 ounces of freshly boiled water and sip up to two quarts of the tea daily. Stir one tablespoon of Swedish Bitters into one cup of tea and drink half before and half after each of the three daily meals.

FATIGUE (SEVERE): If the patient is able to tolerate it, a full bath with an infusion of Thyme may prove amazingly beneficial. The freshening and energizing effects of Thyme are quite remarkable.

FEMALE ORGANS (OVARIES & UTERUS): In any involvement of the female organs, a combination of equal parts of Calendula and Yarrow will prove very beneficial. Use eight heaping teaspoons of the blend for 18 ounces of freshly boiled water. Steep three minutes and strain into a thermos to keep warm. The entire amount should be sipped throughout the day. Before each of the three daily meals, stir one tablespoon of Swedish Bitters into a full cup of the infusion. Take one-half cup before and one-half cup after eating. (Note: Reduce the amount of Swedish Bitters to one teaspoon if the patient has trouble tolerating a full tablespoon.)

Try a daily sitz bath of Yarrow and apply a warm Horsetail poultice to the affected area to draw out the pain. A Swedish Bitters compress will strengthen the treatment.

FLUID RETENTION: If the patient suffers from an accumulation of fluid in the tissues, the recommended daily allotment of tea should be discontinued and five to six cups of an infusion of Horsetail should be substituted. Horsetail purifies and acts as a natural diuretic to reduce bloat. When fluid retention is normalized, discontinue the Horsetail treatment and return to the recommended herbal infusion.

INTESTINES: Please see PANCREAS this chapter.

KIDNEYS: A noted European herbalist recommends a combination of the medicinal herbs for kidney involvement, including cirrhosis of the kidneys. Blend equal proportions of Cleavers, Golden Rod and Yellow Dead Nettle. Use three heaping teaspoons of the blend for every 18 ounces of freshly boiled water (three cups). Cover and steep for four minutes. Stir one teaspoon of Swedish Bitters into the three-cup infusion.

A 20 minute Horsetail sitz bath will help relieve pressure and a warm Horsetail poultice applied to the kidney region overnight greatly aids the patient. During the day, try a Swedish Bitters compress for a period of four hours.

LARYNX/ESOPHAGUS: For problems of the larynx or esophagus, the soothing and coating properties of Mallow have no equal. If it is possible, please make an effort to secure the herb in the fresh state, but dried Mallow can still be effective. Mallow is prepared as a cold infusion (Note: See Chapter 19 for full directions.)

Using one heaping teaspoon of Mallow for every 6 ounces of cold water, prepare 10 cups as the daily allotment and store in a thermos to maintain temperature. Throughout the waking hours, take a total of four cups of the infusion in small sips. The remaining six cups should be used as a deep gargle.

Save the herb residue after preparing the infusion. Add a little hot water and barley flour to the residue and use this mixture as a poultice. Apply to the affected area and wrap warmly for marked relief.

LIVER: To quickly relieve the characteristic shortness of breath which often accompanies both cancer and cirrhosis of the liver, please try one cup of Club Moss tea taken on an empty stomach upon arising and another cup one-half hour before the evening meal. Use one level teaspoon of the herb for every 6 ounces of freshly boiled water.

A Swedish Bitters compress should be applied to the affected area for a period not exceeding four hours during the day. A warm Horsetail poultice should be used for two hours in the morning and again in the afternoon to draw out the pain. Mild Horsetail continues its soothing effect when applied as a poultice overnight.

LUNGS: To help clear the lungs, sip a total of four cups of Yarrow tea throughout the waking hours. In addition, take one cup of an infusion of Horsetail on an empty stomach one-half hour before eating breakfast and another cup one-half hour before the last meal of the day. Try chewing a bit of Calamus Root and washing down the juice with a little Yarrow tea. Spit out the root residue.

If pain is a problem, a warm Horsetail poultice can be applied both to the chest and back overnight. A Swedish Bitters compress should be used for up to four hours during the day as well.

LYMPH: When the lymph glands are involved, the affected areas should be massaged with cold-pressed olive oil prepared with Marjoram or St. John's Wort. Calendula ointment also helps strengthen the body against this condition.

If fresh herbs are available, a pulp of Plantain leaves, Butterbur leaves and Calendula leaves with stems may prove to be a beneficial remedy. These herbs are prepared individually, not as a blend. Wash gently, leave wet, and crush with a wooden rolling pin. Apply the resulting pulp directly to the affected areas on alternate days and allow the patient to decide which herb is most effective.

A blend of three parts Calendula and one part each of Horsetail, Stinging Nettle and Yarrow should be prepared as an infusion. Use one heaping teaspoon of the blended herbs for every 6 ounces of freshly boiled water. A total of two quarts of this tea, taken in small sips during the waking hours of the day, is the recommended daily allotment. Before each of the three daily meals, prepare a full cup of tea and stir in one tablespoon of Swedish Bitters. Take one-half cup before eating and one-half cup after eating. (Note: If the patient cannot tolerate a full tablespoon of Swedish Bitters, reduce this amount to one teaspoon.)

After an operation, the use of Swedish Bitters as a compress or massage aid is said to assist healing. A Horsetail poultice, applied warm mornings and evenings for a period of two hours each application, helps reduce pain and swelling. A Mallow bath will also reduce swelling and is very soothing.

MALE ORGANS (TESTES/PROSTATE): For suggested treatment, please see LYMPH, this chapter. Note: Tight bikini shorts, jeans and trousers have been shown to inhibit the production of sperm. Certain authorities believe there may also be a relationship between the long-term wearing of too-tight trousers and the development of a malignant condition of the male organs.

PANCREAS: Both the pancreas and the intestines are aided by the same regimen. To encourage the appetite and aid the digestive tract, the following herbs are suggested: Blend together two parts Calendula and one part each Stinging Nettle and Yarrow. Use one heaping teaspoon of the blend for each 6 ounces of freshly boiled water. Because up to two quarts daily of this soothing tea are recommended, you may wish to prepare the full amount and keep it warm in a thermos. The patient is advised to take a sip every 15 minutes throughout the waking hours.

Three times daily, stir one tablespoon of Swedish Bitters into one-half cup of this tea and drink one-quarter cup before and one-quarter cup after each of the three main meals of the day. (Note: If a full tablespoon of Swedish Bitters is not easily tolerated, reduce the amount to one teaspoon per one-half cup of tea.)

Six *sips* (not cups) of a cold infusion of Calamus Root is recommended, to be taken as one sip before and one sip after each of the three daily meals. (Please see Chapter 4 for method of preparation.)

To further potentiate the treatment, try a Swedish Bitters compress over the entire abdominal area. A Horsetail poultice acts to relieve pain and may be applied for a two-hour period both mornings and afternoons. Horsetail is mild and soothing and can be left in place overnight.

SKIN: Skin cancer is a growing problem in our sun-worshipping society and is most often surgically removed. Although a natural treatment cannot take the place of competent medical attention, the extracted juice of the Greater Celandine (or Cleavers) can sometimes shrink an affected area, provided the skin remains unbroken.

If the sore has erupted and is supperating, it may be soothed by bathing the area alternately with a warm infusion of Horsetail followed by a cold infusion of Mallow. After this cleansing treatment, dab the edges with Greater Celandine juice and then apply Calendula ointment. Plantain leaves, washed and crushed, may be laid over the open sore. Should the patient be unable to tolerate the crushed Plantain, remove it immediately and again bathe the area with Horsetail and Mallow as directed above. A Horsetail or Mallow compress can be left on overnight and often brings marked relief. (Note: This same treatment will hasten healing if a birthmark, sebaceous cyst, wart or mole has been surgically removed.)

When large areas of the body are affected, try a pain-relieving Horsetail or soothing Mallow (or Thyme) bath. The patient may also benefit by an overnight poultice of crushed Plantain leaves.

A blood-purifying infusion of equal parts of Calendula, Stinging Nettle, Speedwell and Yarrow should be taken daily. Prepare the tea by using one heaping teaspoon of the blended herbs for every 6 ounces of freshly boiled water and drink a total of four cups daily.

STOMACH: Blend together equal parts of Calendula and Stinging Nettle and prepare an infusion using one heaping teaspoon of the blended herbs for every 6 ounces of freshly boiled water. You may wish to store the daily allotment of two quarts in a thermos to retain the heat. Sip throughout the waking hours. In the early stages of stomach involvement, the patient may benefit by adding three to five drops of Wood Sorrel juice to one cup of the infusion. Prepare and drink one cupful every hour.

A Swedish Bitters compress should be applied and left in place for four hours during the day. A warm and soothing Horsetail poultice can be applied to the affected area overnight to ease pain. If the pain is very severe, use a Horsetail poultice for two hours in the morning and again in the afternoon while the patient rests in bed.

THYROID: For an affliction of the thyroid glands, gargle deeply and often with alternate infusions of Cleavers and Mallow. Retain the herb residues after preparing the infusions and mix them individually with warm water and barley flour to prepare a healing poultice. Apply either poultice to the affected area, wrap warmly and leave in place overnight.

During the waking hours, the patient may benefit by relaxing in bed with a warm Horsetail poultice in place for two two-hour periods, once in the morning and again in the afternoon. In addition, apply a Swedish Bitters compress for one four-hour period during the day to hasten healing.

For internal cleansing, an infusion of equal parts of Calendula, Stinging Nettle and Yarrow should be prepared.

TONGUE: The purifying effect of Cleavers aids in any involvement of the tongue. Use one heaping teaspoon of the herb for every 6 ounces of freshly boiled water. Rinse and gargle as deeply as possible with this healing infusion often. The recommended daily allotment is six to eight cups. Sip at least three cups throughout the waking hours and reserve the remaining tea for use as the gargle.

TUMORS (BENIGN & MALIGNANT): A respected European herbalist says Horsetail will arrest the growth of any tumor and can gradually dissolve it. A warm and soothing Horsetail poultice is said to conquer tumors, growths, cysts, ulcers, adenomas, melanomas, papillomas and hematomas. The recommended method of preparation is to place two heaping handfuls of the herb in a collander over boiling water until the mass is soft and hot. Apply directly to the affected area and wrap warmly. This poultice should be used for two hours in the morning and again for two hours in the afternoon. In addition, a Swedish Bitters compress should be used for a period of four hours during the day.

For external tumors, ulcers or growths, washed and crushed Plantain and Cow-Parsnip leaves are reputed to very helpful. Applied regularly and continuously, these fresh-crushed herbs are said to bring improvement within five days and good results after two weeks. The extracted juice of the Wood Sorrel may be rubbed on the affected area as well.

Take one cup of an infusion of Horsetail on an empty stomach one-half hour before breakfast and another cup one-half hour before the evening meal. A combination tea made with three parts Calendula and one part each Stinging Nettle and Yarrow should be prepared. For each cup of tea, three to five drops of extracted Wood Sorrel juice should be added. The patient is directed to take up six cups of this infusion daily at one-hour intervals throughout the waking hours.

Chapter 40
GROWING YOUR OWN HERBS

In days gone by, the traditional place for the household's herb garden was a sunny spot handy to the kitchen door. If you have even a tiny yard that receives sun during at least part of the day, you can still easily grow a few of the medicinal herbs. We have provided growing requirements and brief guidelines for planting the herbs detailed in each chapter, and you will receive in-depth instruction from the source where you purchase either bedding plants or seed packets.

But, in today's modern world, many of us live in patio homes, rented apartments, or high-rises without a bit of earth to call our own. Fortunately, herbs lend themselves nicely to indoor gardening or a combination of indoor and outdoor gardening. For instance, small potted herbs will flourish on tiered shelves in a sunny city window without ever a breath of fresh air. If you have a balcony or patio, large pots can be moved outside in the summer to catch the direct rays of the sun and brought inside for shelter against winter's icy winds.

One particularly attractive method of cultivating a variety of herbs in a small space you might consider is the traditional 'strawberry pot' or 'strawberry barrel.'

Many nurseries stock various sizes of what are termed 'strawberry pots.' These pots, made of terra cotta clay, have a number of 'pockets' opening into the interior which protrude slightly from the rounded outside of the pot. As a rule of thumb, strawberry pots cost around $1.00 per pocket in most areas. They range in size from a small one with three pockets (around $3.00) to the giant size with one-hundred openings (around $100.00). These pots are very attractive when planted with a selection of herbs tucked into their pockets. The silvery-gray, myriad shades of green and tiny flowering varieties of the different herbs are showcased against the deep, rusty orange of the terra cotta.

The 'strawberry (or herb) barrel' follows the same principle and can be easily made at home.

Thirty-gallon whiskey casks suitable for transforming into herb barrels can be obtained from many nurseries and distilleries. Depending on your source, a full-size cask will cost anywhere from $20.00 to

$50.00 and will provide a home for up to 100 herbs. Half-size, three-quarter and even one-quarter size barrels are also readily available. Because they have been cut and will not have lids, you will need to provide a metal bottom to contain the soil if you wish to convert a cut size into a small herb barrel.

After you have secured a suitable cask, the next step is to drill holes two inches in diameter and four inches apart (in every direction) in a pleasing pattern around the circumference of the barrel and in the lid. Drill a series of small holes around the outside circumference of the lid to provide for watering. Five or six two-inch holes will probably be all the lid will accommodate for planting. Also drill a small center hole in the lid for watering. If you don't have a drill or the space to work, ask the nursery to do it for you or prevail on a friend with a home workshop. You're certain to find someone who thinks your herb barrel is a fascinating project. Promise them some herb wine or a packet of dried medicinal herbs as a barter.

Once you have the barrel prepared, the next step is to provide a suitable growing medium for the herbs with a core of small rocks to insure good drainage. A porous soil mix which holds water and nutrients, but which drains quickly, is required. Ask the nursery man for a good comercial potting soil which is light, uniform in texture, disease-free (sterilized), and with a balanced nutrient content. If you wish, you may mix up your own potting soil by following the 'recipe' included in this chapter.

Begin preparing the barrel by pouring soil into it around the outside curve and fill it inward to the center core of rocks. This will be four to six inches, depending on the diameter of your barrel. You may wish to dampen the growing medium to help keep it where you want it and to prevent it from spilling out the drilled holes, but don't worry if the soil and rocks intermingle where they meet. Continue building up the soil around the outside and rock in the center until the entire barrel has been well filled.

If you happen to have a muscle-man handy, it would help hasten the inevitable settling to lift the barrel a few inches and let it drop several times. Otherwise, water well and wait a few days before planting to allow gravity to take care of the job. If you plant before everything has had time to settle, you may find your tender young herbs out of position and hanging by the neck (until dead) out their respective holes.

Consider the water requirements of your herbs when positioning them in the barrel. The plants which require a lot of moisture should be positioned in the lid itself or the top half of the barrel. Those which require less moisture will be quite happy farther down the barrel. Generally speaking, most herbs are drought-resistant. However, container-grown herbs correctly potted in a good porous mixture with good drainage can be watered freely with little danger of root-rot.

HOW TO PREPARE A SUITABLE POTTING SOIL: As outlined earlier in this chapter, a good potting soil for herbs (or any container grown plant) should be light in texture and porous enough to provide good drainage and an adequate oxygen supply. It should hold a lot of water and nutrients without becoming compacted around tender roots, but it should not hold moisture so long that root rot can develop. The pH and nutrient content should be in balance and the mix must be disease-free to insure healthy plants. Preparing your own potting mixture can result in significant savings, but only if you require a large quantity. Otherwise, your best buy is a bag of a good quality blend.

This recipe will yield two bushels of good potting soil.

MIX TOGETHER WELL:
1 bushel sphagnum peat moss (milled)
1 bushel perlite or vermiculite (horticultural-grade)
10 tablespoons limestone (powdered)
5 tablespoons phosphate
2 tablespoons potassium nitrate
1 teaspoon iron chelate

If you are planning a small trial-planting of herbs, indoors or out, we suggest you consider the premiere medicinal herbs: Calendula, Chamomile, Comfrey, Dandelion, Echinacea, Horsetail, Mallow, Speedwell, Stinging Nettle, St. John's Wort and Yarrow. See the appropriate chapters for full information on their respective properties, characteristics and growing requirements.

Once the herbs on your window ledge, in your garden, barrel or strawberry pot, are well established, you will be rewarded with fresh cuttings of your favorite medicinals just about any time of the year. In addition, their subtle colors enhance any corner where they are placed and their faint fragrances will freshen the air just as they did in medieval times, as long as you select wisely. Don't forget that some growing herbs have a distinctly unpleasant scent, especially in a closed room.

APPENDIX

SOURCES OF HERBS AND HERB PRODUCTS

CALIFORNIA

Herbs of Mexico
3859 Whittier Blvd.
Los Angeles, CA 90023
Tel. (213) 221-0064
(Herbs from all over the world)

Kitazawa Seed Co.
356 W. Taylor St.
San Jose, CA 95110
Tel. (408) 292-4420
(Seeds)

Lhasa Karnak Herb Co.
2513 Telegraph Ave.
Berkeley, CA 94704
Tel. (415) 548-0380
(Herbs, teas, spices)

Nature's Herb Company
281 Ellis St.
San Francisco, CA 94102
Tel. (415) 474-2756
(Herbs, herbal preparations)

Organic Foods & Gardens
4177 W. 3rd St.
Los Angeles, CA 90040
Tel. (213) 386-1440
(Herbs, etc.)

CONNECTICUT

Capriland's Herb Farm
Silver St.
Coventry, CT 06238
Tel. (203) 742-7244
(Herbs)

IDAHO

Lewiston Health Food Center
861 Main
Lewiston, ID 83501
Tel. (208) 799-3100
(Herbs)

ILLINOIS

Dr. Michael's Herb Products
5109 North Western Ave.
Chicago, IL 60625
Tel. (312) 271-7738
(Herb products)

Kramer's Health Food Store
29 East Adams St.
Chicago, IL 60603
Tel. (312) 922-0077
(Herbs)

INDIANA

Indiana Botanic Gardens, Inc.
Box 5
Hammond, IN 46325
Tel. (219) 931-2480
(Herbs, herb preparations, gums, oils, resins)

Moses J. Troyer
Lone Organic Farm
Route 1, Box 58
Millersburg, IN 46543
Tel. (219) 642-3385
(Herbs)

KENTUCKY

Ferry-Morse Seed Co.
Box 200
Fulton, KY 42041
Tel. (502) 472-3400
(Herbs, seeds)

MAINE

Conley's Garden Center
Boothbay Harbor, ME 04538
Tel. (207) 633-5020
(Wildflowers, ferns, garden plants)

MARYLAND

Carroll Gardens
P.O. Box 310
East Main St.
Westminster, Md 21157
Tel. 1-800-638-6334
(Herbs)

NEW JERSEY

Le Jardin du Gourmet
Box 245
Ramsey, NJ 07446
Tel. (201) 891-2070
(Herbs, spices, seeds)

NEW YORK

Kalustyan Orient Export
Trading Corp.
123 Lexington Ave.
New York, NY 10016
Tel. (212) 685-3416
(Herbs, spices)

Kiehl Pharmacy
109 Third Ave.
New York, NY 10003
Tel. (212) 475-3400
(Herbs, spices)

H. Roth & Son
1577 First Ave.
New York, NY 10028
Tel. (212) 734-1110
(212) 535-2322
(Herbs, spices)

NORTH CAROLINA

Wilcox Drug Co., Inc.
P.O. Box 391
Boone, NC 28607
Tel. (704) 264-3615
(Herbs)

OREGON

Nichols Garden Nursery
1190 North Pacific Highway
Albany, OR 97321
Tel. (503) 928-9280
(Herbs, spices, seeds, plants)

PENNSYLVANIA

Haussman's Pharmacy
6th & Girard Ave.
Philadelphia, PA 19127
Tel. (215) 627-2143
(Herbs, mixtures, oil, gums)

Penn Herb Company
603 N. 2nd St.
Philadelphia, PA 19123
Tel. (215) 925-3336
(Herbs)

Tatra Herb Company
222 Grove St.
Morrisville, PA 19067
Tel. (215) 722-5305
(Herbs)

RHODE ISLAND

Greene Herb Gardens
Greene, RI 02827
Tel. (401) 397-3652
(Fresh and dried herbs, teas, seeds)

Meadowbrook Herb Garden
Route 138
Wyoming, RI 02898
Tel. (401) 539-7603 or
1-800-253-5005
(Herbs, herb products, spices)

TENNESSEE

Savage Farm Nursery
Box 125
McMinnville, TN 37110
Tel. (615) 668-8902
(Wildflowers, garden plants)

VERMONT

Putney Nursery, Inc.
Box 13
Putney, VT 05346
Tel. (802) 387-5577
(Wildflowers)

Vermont Country Store
Weston, VT 05161
Tel. (802) 824-3184
(Herbs, spices, condiments,
grains)

WASHINGTON

Cedarbrook Herb Farm
Route 1, Box 1047
Sequim, WA 98382
Tel. (206) 683-7733
(Herb plants)

WISCONSIN

Northwestern Processing Co.
217 North Broadway
Milwaukee, WI 53202
Tel. (414) 276-1031
(Herbs, teas, nuts, spices)

Olds Seed Co.
Box 1069
Madison, WI 53701
Tel. (608) 221-9877
(Seeds)

CANADA

World-Wide Herb Ltd.
11 St. Catherine St. East
Montreal 129, Quebec
Tel. (514) 842-1838
(Herbs)

For Your Convenience

Although most of the herbs and products discussed in *The Miracle Healing Power Through Nature's Pharmacy* are available in major health food stores nationwide, you may sometimes have trouble locating a particular item that seems just right for you.

When that time comes, or if you just plain prefer armchair shopping convenience, we suggest you request a catalog from *New Dimensions Distributors.* This forward-thinking organization carries many hard-to-find health-related herbs, products and devices. You'll like the friendly staff, toll-free ordering, prompt service, and their selection of quality products. Here's their address:

INDEX

A

B

B (cont'd.)

C

D

E

F

G

H

I

J

K

L

M

N

O

P

Q

R

S

T

U

V

W

Y

Z

Other Outstanding Books On Health And Natural Healing From Fischer Publishing

How To Survive In The Hospital
by Joan Haas-Unger, RN

In an easy-to-read style, this book tells how hospitals, doctors and nurses work . . . but more important, it discusses how to make them work for you! A small sample of the topics covered in this landmark book: "How to pick the best doctor, how to get pain medication when you need it, what you need to know about surgery . . . your options may surprise you. How to avoid unnecessary tests, how to prevent bedsores . . . constipation . . . urinary tract infections . . . boredom . . . and a host of other common problems." You'll read in vivid detail why being a passive patient is asking for trouble in today's fast-paced pressurized hospitals. The perfect consumer guide to hospitalization.

ISBN 0-915421-06-2 $12.95

Hidden Secrets Of Super Perfect Health At Any Age
Book II—*by William L. Fischer*

Contains never-before-published health-related information with an incredible number of alternatives for treating everything from cancer to insomnia, from prostate problems to male impotence, from varicose veins to migraine headaches. Brings hope to sufferers of colitis, arthritis, bronchitis, asthma, heart problems, poor circulation and more. 288 pages.

ISBN 0-915421-05-4 $14.95

The Miracle Healing Power Of Chelation Therapy
by Dr. Morton Walker

Dr. Walker has compiled the most impressive book every written on Chelation Therapy . . . plus everything you've wanted to know about this miracle treatment for hardening of the arteries, diabetes, stroke, senility, impotence, glaucoma, Alzheimer's Disease, and many other common arterial and degenerative diseases including numerous documented case histories and names of chelating physicians.

ISBN 0-915421-00-3 $18.95

How To Fight Cancer And Win
by William L. Fischer

It clearly spells out real cancer preventives and cures, many never before published, with strong scientific documentation and stories of miraculous cures. They are all presented in a concise easy-to-understand style. You can put this vast knowledge into practice to insure that this deadly disease never strikes home.

ISBN 0-915421-07-0 $14.95

Shipping and handling—$2.00; for each additional book—$ .50

fischer publishing one fischer square box 368 canfield, ohio 44406